The
POWER
of Your
SPINE

How Back Strength and
Posture Pilots the Entire Body

By

Tracy L. Markley. C.P.T.

Certified Fitness & Biomechanics Specialist

TABLE OF CONTENTS

FOREWORD
BY DR. EVAN OSAR

If your goal is to retire and enjoy the proverbial fruits of your labor, you will need to invest in your financial future. You meet with a financial planner who helps you understand, manage, and navigate your portfolio, so that you and your loved ones are well provided for when you retire.

Unfortunately, many of us know far more about our financial status – and even our automobiles – than we understand about our body. Very few of us have invested the same amount of time and attention in our health and well-being as we have in our financial futures. This is unfortunate, because the reality for most of our society is that they will spend a great deal of their retirement –

time, money, and energy – going to doctors to deal with the years of neglecting their body.

Muscle and joint pain are the leading causes of disability in our older adult population. One in three older individuals will fall and experience a significant injury and/or require hospitalization as a result. Muscle weakness and tightness as well as poor posture and overall deconditioning are the leading causes of these falls. On a larger scale, joint and muscle pain, along with tightness, weakness, and inevitably, contribute to the lack of physical activity and the rapid deterioration of one's health. These issues contribute to further disability as well as more time, money, and energy required to manage these conditions.

However, it does not have to be this way and there is a simple solution. That solution is:

Develop a more optimal and efficient strategy for posture and movement.

When you develop more optimal and efficient posture and movement habits, you will improve your strength and stability. When you develop more optimal and efficient posture and movement habits, you will improve your flexibility and experience less tightness and discomfort. And when you develop more optimal and efficient posture and movement habits, you will experience increased health and vitality.

Tracy has created a resource, a blueprint if you will call it this, for understanding your body. Just like a blueprint is a guide for building your house, this book is your blueprint for developing your foundation for posture and movement. Through her easy-to-understand illustrations and descriptions, Tracy will help you understand your joints, muscles, and how they contribute to posture, balance, and movement. More importantly, she will help you incorporate this information into a simple strategy for improving your posture, strength, balance, flexibility, and overall well-being.

Invest in yourself and take control of your health and well-being. Read this book, and more importantly, apply the information. See what a difference it can make in your life.

Yours in health,

Dr. Evan Osar
Developer of the *Integrative Movement System*™
Physician, Author, Speaker

INTRODUCTION

J.A. Mastropaolo wrote so wonderfully in his book, *Kinesiology for the Public Schools*:

Muscles create the movement that maintains life. The breathing muscles power the air into and out of the lungs, where oxygen goes into the blood. The heart muscle Powerfully pumps the blood's oxygen to every cell in the body. To stay alive, the body needs oxygen more than anything else. That is why everyone needs to know how to maintain powerful breathing muscles and a powerful heart. The only way to maintain a powerful heart and breathing muscles is to exercise the body's skeletal muscles.

A healthy, strong back and posture lead to a stronger walking gait, better balance, and healthier shoulders, hips, knees, ankles, and feet joints. For the legs and arms to perform at their best for everyday activities and sports, the spine and back muscles must be strong to help the body sustain proper and functional posture for power in movements and to remain injury-free.

Movement begins at the spine. It is important to learn the muscles of the spine and back and how they all lead to movements throughout the body. A healthy spine can move in seven different directions. These different directions lead to the movement of the limbs in everyday activities, including walking.

Poor posture can cause neuromuscular communications to be compromised. If you or someone you know is in any kind of rehab or in stroke recovery, poor posture will limit recovery.

In this book, I bring you anatomy illustrations of many of the muscles of the spine and the back. I share basic and some complex knowledge of the important job of each muscle. As you gain more understanding of your muscles and movements, you will be able to bring what you have learned into your physical therapy and exercise routines to help you gain greater strength in your spine, back, and core. This will lead to overall strength and balance, which can lead to fewer injuries.

The Core, has become a cliché to many. When people speak of the core, they often think of having six-pack muscles or having a flat belly. People are told by friends and doctors with back pain to strengthen their core, but they are given no concrete knowledge of what that really means. Many are left not knowing how to achieve this and/or trying to achieve it by exercising on machines and/or basic floor abdominal exercises.

When you understand more about the muscles and movements of your own body, it will help you have a stronger body, stay injury-free, maintain your balance and stability, heal from injuries, and understand your rehabilitation exercises. At any age, you will be better at sports and stronger at performing your everyday activities.

With all my books, I try to keep it simple and to the point to make it easy to follow along. As you read this book, please understand that the muscles are not shared in the exact order they layer in the body.

This book is also a great resource for any student that needs to study anatomy for school, physical therapy, fitness, Pilates, and yoga certifications and more. It is a great resource to take along to your physical therapists, personal trainers, fitness professionals, massage therapists, chiropractors, and doctors. This can help you and your professionals work together to help you build a stronger, more functional, and healthier body.

CHAPTER 1

THE SPINAL BONES

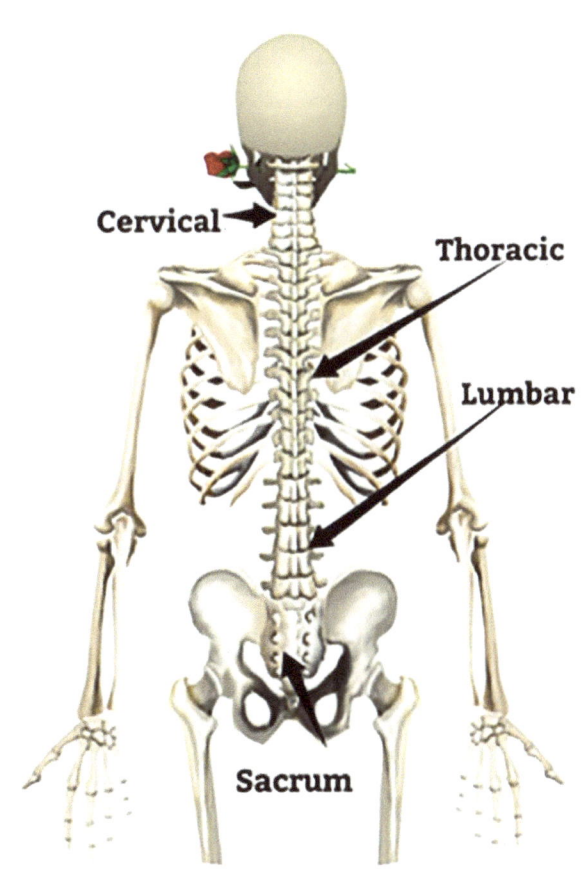

The spine is made up of:

Seven cervical vertebrae,

Twelve thoracic vertebrae,

Five lumbar vertebrae,

The sacrum; which is five vertebrae fused together.

At the bottom of the sacrum is the "coccyx," which is known as the tail bone.

One of my college teachers taught me a fun way to remember the number of vertebrae that we have:

We eat breakfast at 7:00, lunch at 12:00, and dinner at 5:00.

CHAPTER 2

THE SPINAL CORD

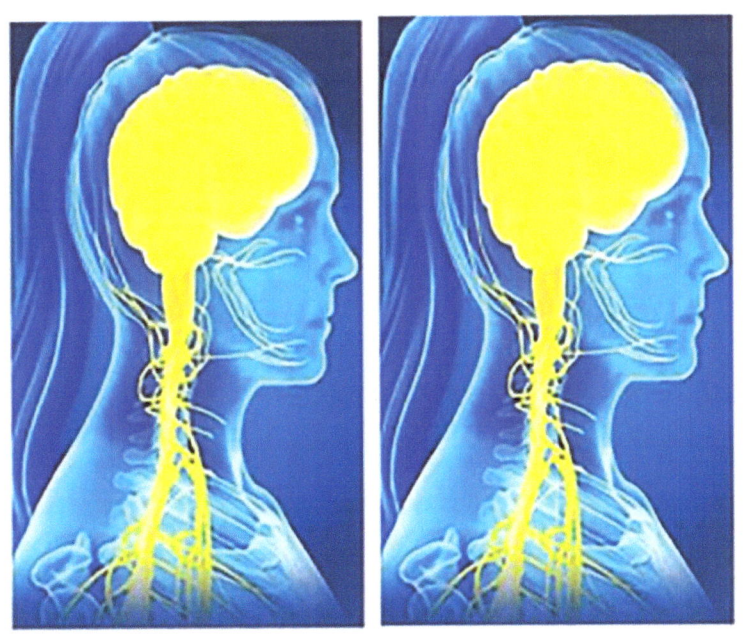

The spinal cord is the communicator between the brain and the body. It carries messages that allow us to move and feel sensations. Spinal nerve cells, also called neurons, carry messages to and from the spinal cord. Spinal nerve roots branch out of the spinal cord in pairs to reach each side of the body. The messages leave the spinal cord through the openings in the vertebrae. Each nerve has a specific job for a movement in the body as well as the physical feeling or perception of something that happens to or that meets the body. When the musculoskeletal system is in poor posture, neuromuscular communication will be compromised.

The spinal cord coordinates and controls the activities of our bodies. The brain and spinal cord (spinal column) together are known as the central nervous system. The brain is covered by the skull and the spinal cord is covered by the vertebrae. They both are covered by a protective membrane called meninges. The stronger the posture becomes, the stronger the entire body becomes.

It is a proven fact that all systems in the body function better if the body is in proper posture. This means the nervous system work better if the body maintains a proper posture. This begins in the spine.

Poor posture can provoke pain by constricting blood vessels and nerves. If you or someone you know is having neurological challenges or is recovering from a stroke, the posture of the spine can play an essential role in rehabbing and healing the whole body. Our bodies were made to move. When the muscles and bones around the messaging system are strong and functioning at their best, the spinal cord and messaging system of the brain and body (which is responsible for movement) will also function better. I know this from experience in working with those who have neurological challenges. As the client's posture gets stronger and balanced, the movement and sensations to the limbs will also become stronger.

Extra facts:

The central nervous system is the brain and the spinal column.

There are meninges that cover and protect the central nervous system. The meninges are three layers of protective tissues that protect the brain and spinal cord. These three layers are called Dura Mater, Arachoid Mater, and Pia Mater that surround the

Neuroaxixs. The meninges of the brain and spinal column are linked through the magnum foramen.

Neuroaxis is also known as the Neuraxis.

CHAPTER 3

THE SEVEN DIRECTIONS OF SPINAL MOVEMENT

The human spine can move in seven directions. These movements Include:

1. Forward flexion of the spine – Forward bending.

2. Backward extension of the spine – Backward bending.

3. Flexing sideways to one side of the body. Lateral bending to one side.

4. Extending back to the center of the body after flexing to one side and lateral bending to the other side.

5. Rotation of the spine to one direction. Rotation to the right and left.

6. Rotation of the spine from one direction back to the center and to the other side.

7. Axial extension - Moving from a slouching position to sitting up tall. Extending the spine straight to the sky into good posture.

The more you understand how the parts of your anatomy work together, the better you can help your body function and become stronger.

Spinal Flexion and Extension

Bending (flexing) forward and bending (extending) backward

Below are extreme spinal flexion and spinal extension. As you learn more about the movements and muscles, you will understand that a small movement in these directions is still considered spinal flexion and extension. Spinal extension includes: straightening back up from bending forward and extending backward. My angles in these pictures may seem exaggerated or farther than you can go, but that is okay. It is done to give a visual of the movements, so you can connect to the movements you do in your everyday life.

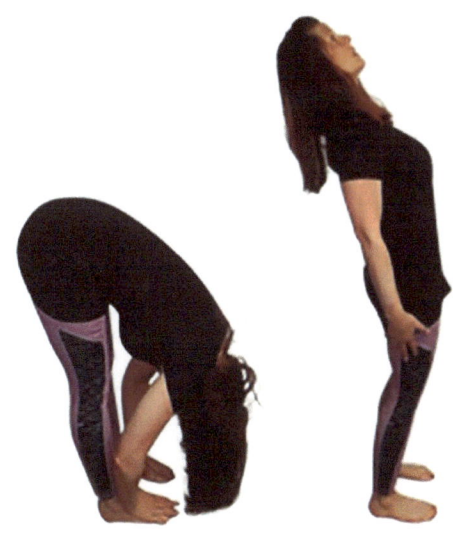

Lateral Spinal Flexion and Extension

Bending the torso right and left

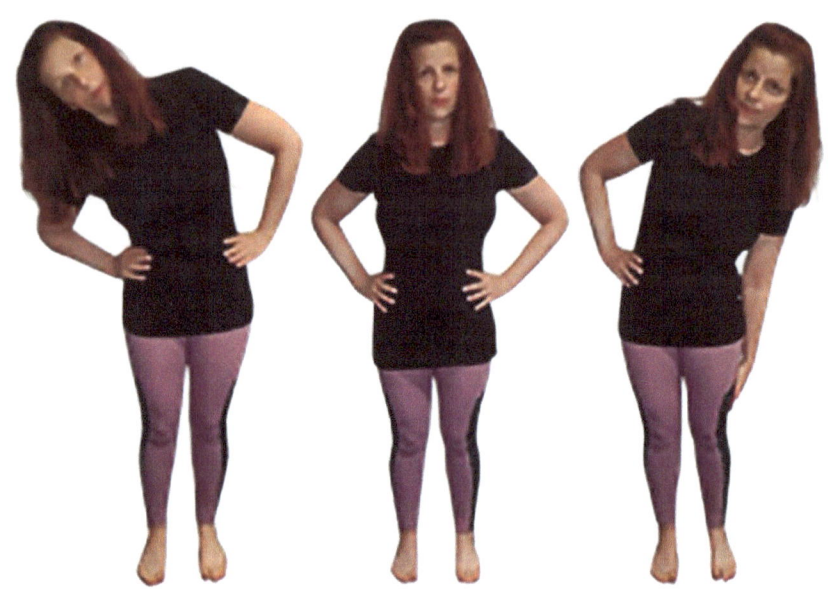

Lateral flexion to one direction and lateral extension to bring the body back to an upright position.

Extra Tips:

If you have osteopenia, osteoporosis, weakness, or injury in your spine, you should always support your lateral flexion, as you see in the pictures above. The hand is touching the waist or the side of the leg on the side of the body it is flexing towards.

Spinal Rotation

Spinal Rotation Outward – rotating as if looking away from the body.

Spinal Rotation Inward – bringing the rotation movement back in from rotating outward.

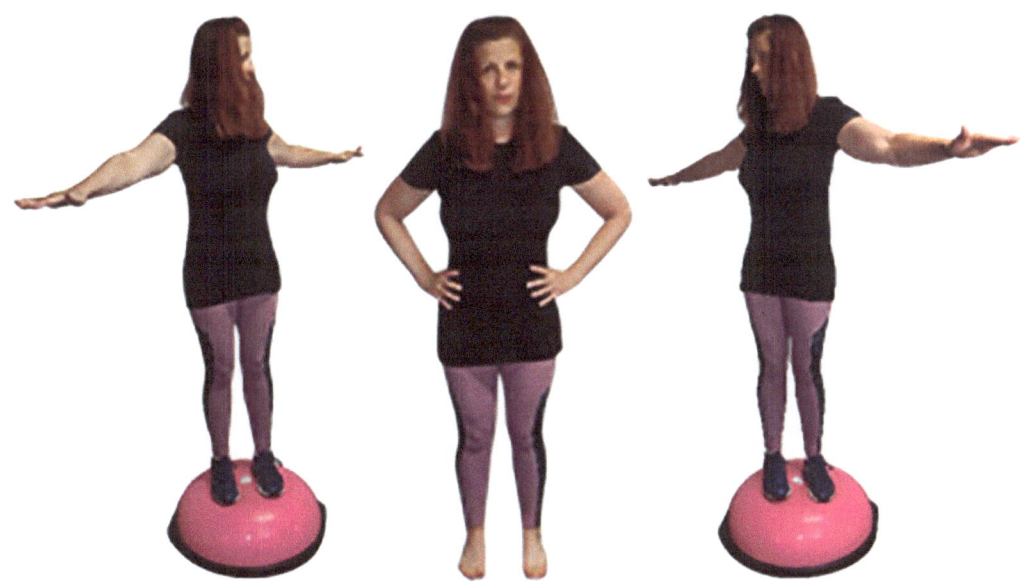

Remember in spinal rotation: If you have an injury, rotation is not always the best movement to begin with to strengthen the spine and back. If you have an injury in or near your spine and you are uncertain where to begin, have a therapist direct you properly for your safety and to avoid future or permanent injury.

One of the most common injuries of the spine is spinal flexion and spinal rotation at the same time. This happens often when someone is picking up a box and staying bent over and then twists the spine to place or finish lifting the box. Proper posture is essential.

Axial Extension

Axial Extension position is the movement of going from a slouching position to a sitting up or standing tall position. This movement extends upwards, lengthening the spine up (taller) into proper posture. Here are a few examples:

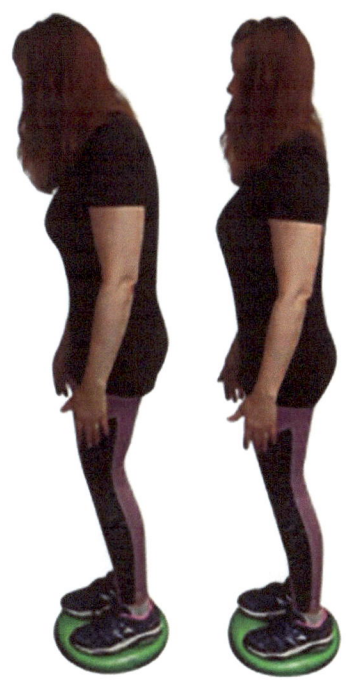

An important tip while working on posture and balance is that while standing and/or walking, keep your eyes looking forward. Your body follows where your eyes look. If you look or face down, the body will try to follow, as in the first picture above. It will keep you in poor posture.

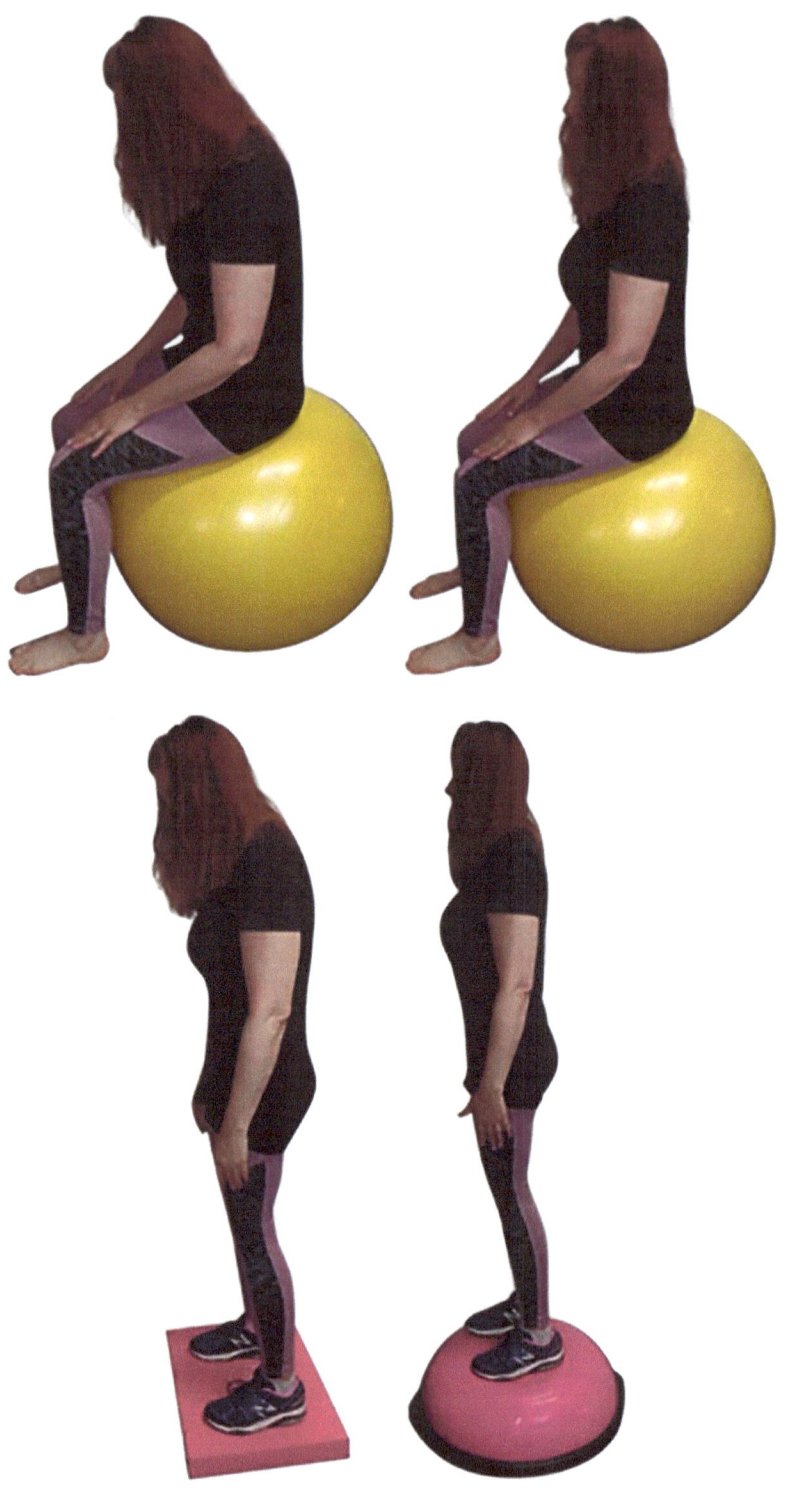

The reason I shared different variations of the slouching and the Axial Extension is because a large percentage of people in the world have some sort of back pain or discomfort. Poor posture is just one of the reasons for this. Poor posture will limit you from moving properly, strongly, and safely.

Keep these visuals in mind as you learn about the spine and back muscles that I share in this book. You will notice that you are either sitting, standing, or moving throughout the day. It will become clear quickly why you may be experiencing pain. Poor posture does not only have a negative effect on the back, but it also affects the shoulders, arms, elbows, wrists, fingers, hips, pelvic, legs, knees, ankles, feet, and toes. It also has a negative effect on the fascia throughout the body. Poor posture creates faulty movements with the joints in your everyday activities and your everyday non- activities such as sitting.

This is very important to understand if you are in any sort of rehabilitation from surgeries, injuries and challenges such as learning to stand and walk. This would include stroke survivors and brain injury populations. Although I am not a physical therapist, 75% of my clients are in some sort of rehabilitation. I work with many stroke survivors and clients, needing to regain their balance and stability and learning the skills to feel safe in everyday movements and walking.

The clients who work on their posture everywhere they go, not just when they are with me, get the best results.

Here is an example of a client who is learning to walk again after a stroke. In the first picture, you can see how his hips are off to one side and his posture is poor. When he tries to stand up from that position, it does not work. He is attempting to start up from sitting to standing in a faulty and weak functional position.

In the second picture, you can see how his hips, legs, knees, and feet are in a good position to move from sitting to standing. It may not be easy to see in these photos, but I recently had him change his sitting cushion in his wheelchair. In the first picture, he is sitting on a cushion that has no support for his hips and spine, and he just sank into it. In the second picture, he is sitting on a cushion that is made to give his hip and spine support in computer chairs. Switching the seat cushions greatly helped him to maintain a proper seating position needed to aid the functional movement needed to stand and walk.

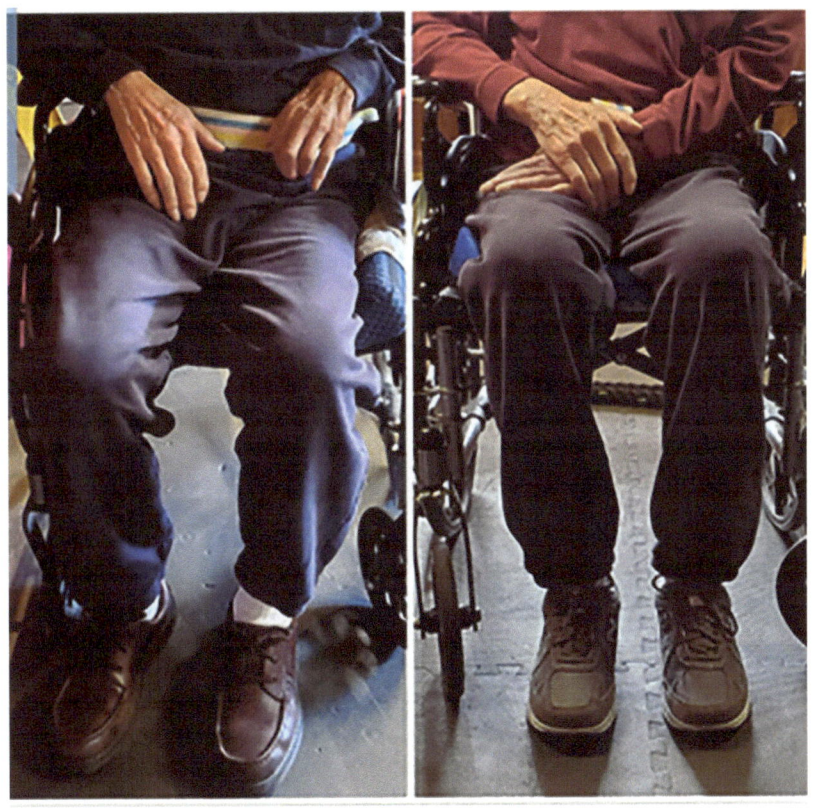

The position the body spends more time in is usually the position the body will try to use for everyday movements, such as the example in the picture above. If he sits for hours a day in a poor spine and hip position, the body will try to use that position for all activities. The communication between the brain and spinal cord can be compromised. If he sits upright in good posture with his hips positioned properly, the body will be stronger to move properly when needed as well as the communication between the spinal cord and brain will be better.

Now, look at just the
low spine area and pelvic bones.

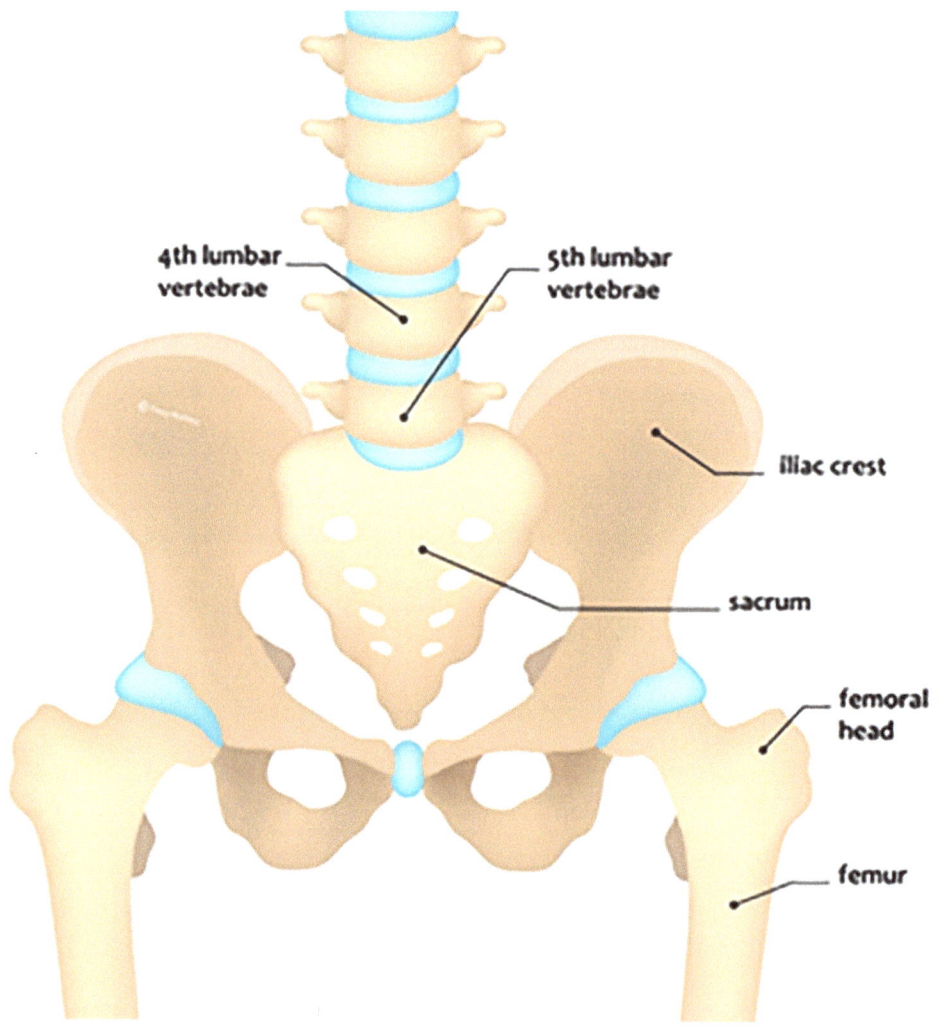

4th lumbar vertebrae

5th lumbar vertebrae

iliac crest

sacrum

femoral head

femur

Here is a visual to help you picture how the muscles and spine connect. FYI, the sciatic nerve comes through the 4th and 5th lumbar vertebrae. More on that later.

NOTES

CHAPTER 4

MUSCLES OF
THE SPINE AND BACK

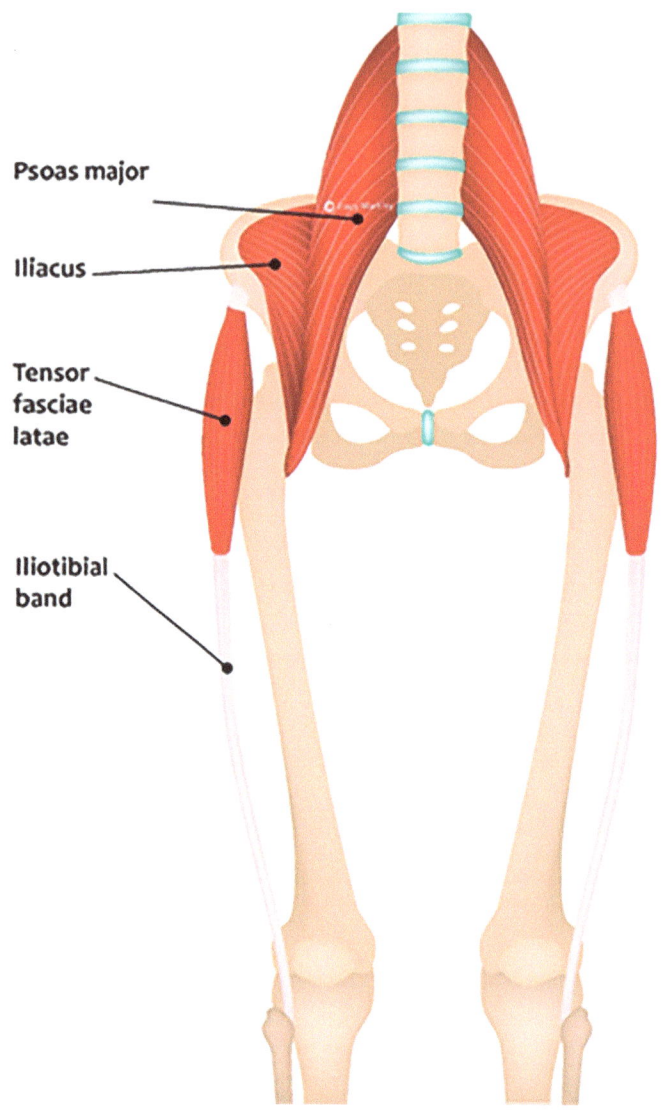

Psoas major

Iliacus

Tensor
fasciae
latae

Iliotibial
band

If you have read my first three books, some of what I share about the "**psoas**" may sound familiar. The **psoas muscle** is an extremely important muscle located in the center of the body. It lies deep underneath the transverse abdominal muscle. It is a deep back muscle. It is the only spine muscle that directly attaches to the legs. The psoas muscle is the only muscle in the back that crosses over the hips and attaches at the front of the body. It attaches at the last thoracic vertebrae and to four of the five lumbar vertebrae and at the femur, the upper thigh bone. It is also the bridge between the hips and the back. Often, it is referred to as the iliopsoas. This is when the psoas and the iliacus muscles are grouped together.

Fascia has numerous attachments to the trunk, spine, pelvis, and hips. Fascia attaches to several muscles including the diaphragm, quadratus lumborum, transverse abdominal, pelvic floor, and iliacus.

The movements of the psoas muscles are:

Flexion and lateral rotation of the thigh. This means lifting the knee towards the chest and rotating it out open to the side. When the feet are fixed to the ground, it is bilateral contraction (meaning both sides working together) and helps perform trunk flexion. If only one side, it is unilateral contraction (meaning just one side), and it rotates the pelvic and trunk to the opposite directions.

If the abdominal muscles are weak, the psoas tries to perform the work of the abdominal. If the psoas is short, weak, and/or tight, it will be difficult to hold the body in an upright position with the shoulders stacked over the hips. If a person exercises in this position, it will build poor functioning skills.

The psoas muscle works closely with the diaphragm. The diaphragm is the main muscle for breathing. The psoas is the main muscle for walking. The psoas attaches at the lumbar spine and the crura of the diaphragm attach there as well. The crura (plural for crus), are two fibroelastic bands that come up from the lumbar vertebrae and insert into the central tendon of the diaphragm. There is one on the left side and one on the right side. Together, they perform a muscle contraction. A person must walk and breathe at the same time. The psoas and the diaphragm must be strong for movement and walking.

Extra tip:

Visualize the psoas as sitting in poor posture. For those learning to stand and walk again, like the man in the previous pictures, sitting properly helps the psoas maintain a balance between both sides and the pull on the vertebra as well as making it work properly for everyday movements.

The following images are modified and adapted from The Psoas Solution: by Dr. Evan Osar and published by Lotus Publishing.

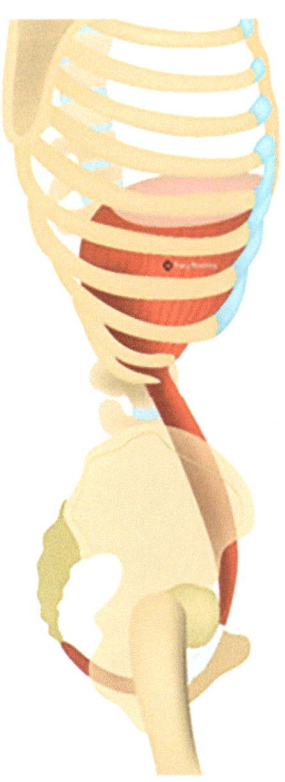

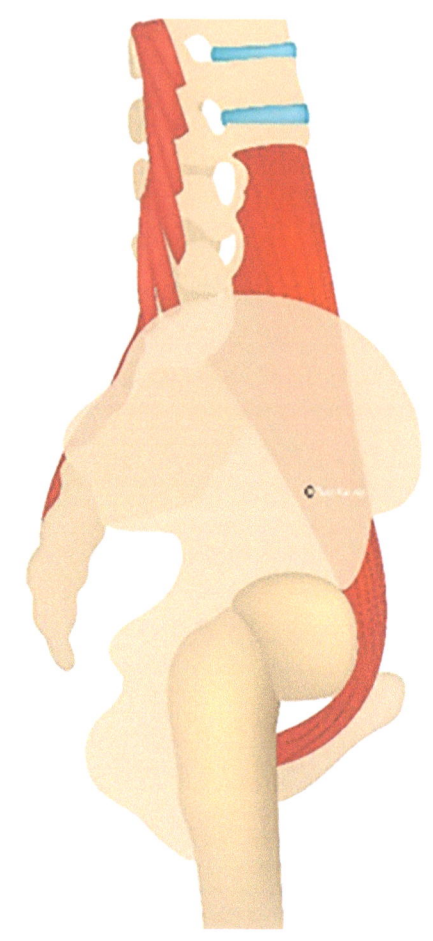

In the first illustration, you see a side view of the diaphragm and the psoas muscles. The second illustration is a partial side view of the multifidus and the psoas muscles.

These are great images from Dr. Evan Osar, which allow us to learn more about the proper movement of the human body. The trunk must be strong to help hold the diaphragm up in proper position, so the psoas can work fully and safely. If the upper body and diaphragm are hunched over and where the psoas fascia and diaphragm fascia blend, that area will be out of natural placement, leading to faulty movement, weakness, injury, and pain. This will affect walking, standing, and everyday movements.

Multifidus Muscle

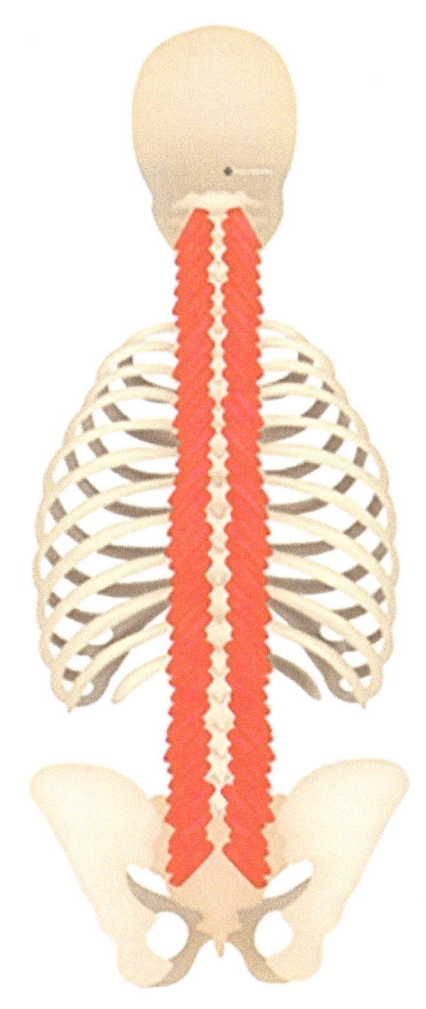

The **multifidus** muscles are small but powerful muscles. It is the main stabilizing muscle of the spine. This muscle takes pressure off the vertebral discs, so that the body weight can be distributed throughout the spine. If this is weak, you will also have weakness in the lower back. The **multifidus** begins to activate before the body moves to protect the spine. It is part of the stabilizing system in the body. The multifidus is also one of the muscles in the spine that extends, abducts, adducts, and rotates the spine. To gain better balance, this muscle must be strong. Performing various exercises combined with the Swiss ball, balance disc, and BOSU® ball will help gain a stronger multifidus. Better posture leads to better balance.

To help make these easier to understand, when we bend over from the spine (rounding the spine) that is called spinal flexion. When we are pulling the spine from flexed position back up to being upright, this movement is called spinal extension, also known as Axial Extension. Flexion is when a muscle brings two joints together. Extension is bringing the two joints farther apart. For example, when we flex our arm while performing a bicep curl exercise, that is flexion, and as you extend the arm back out straight, that is extension.

The small muscles near the vertebrae need to be activated harmoniously. These are postural muscles. Exercising on an unstable surface, such as the Swiss ball, balance disc, and the BOSU® ball, stimulates the central nervous system, which is the brain and the spinal cord. It strengthens muscles and ligaments, as well as activating and strengthening all the small muscles along the spinal column.

The **multifidus muscle**, **transverse abdominal muscle**, **diaphragm,** and the **pelvic floor muscles** are all on the same neuromuscular loop. This means that it is best if all these muscles are functioning properly; each needs to perform its job individually <u>and</u> as a team. Stated a bit more complicated: It means a sequential, segmental neuromuscular stimulation with closed-loop feedback. If the transverse muscle is weak, the pelvic floor, the multifidus, and the diaphragm cannot gain proper strength to perform their jobs in a healthy, functioning body.

These muscles are not all considered to be back muscles, but they all must be strong in order for the back muscles to be strong.

Spinal Rotator Muscles

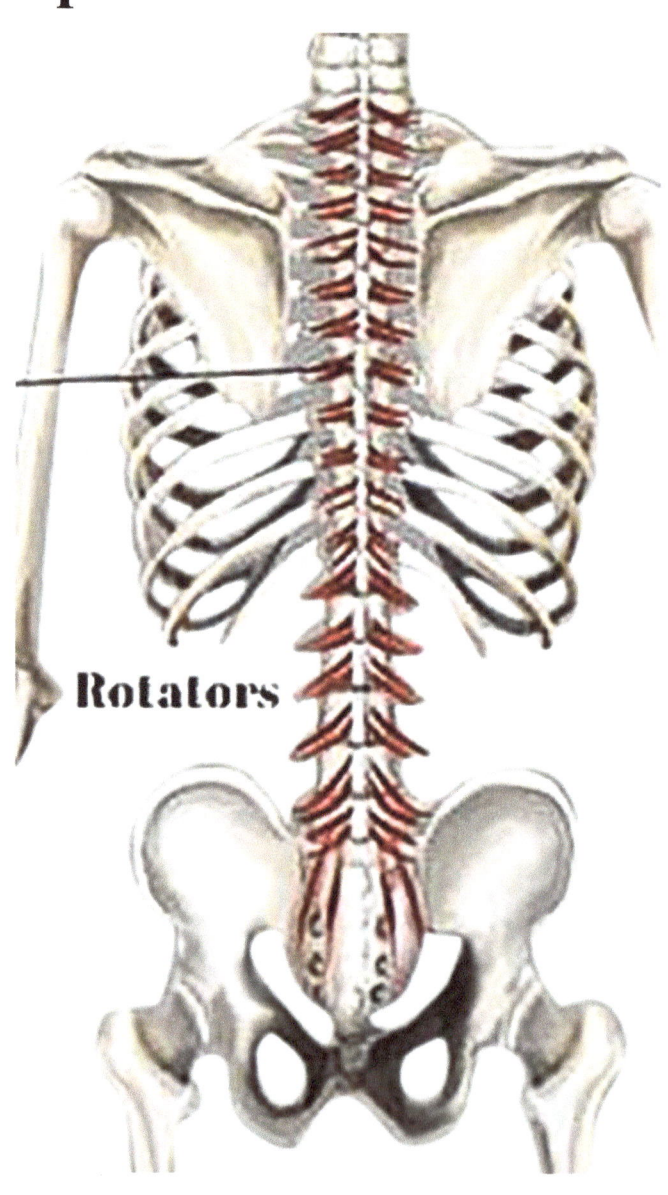

Rotators

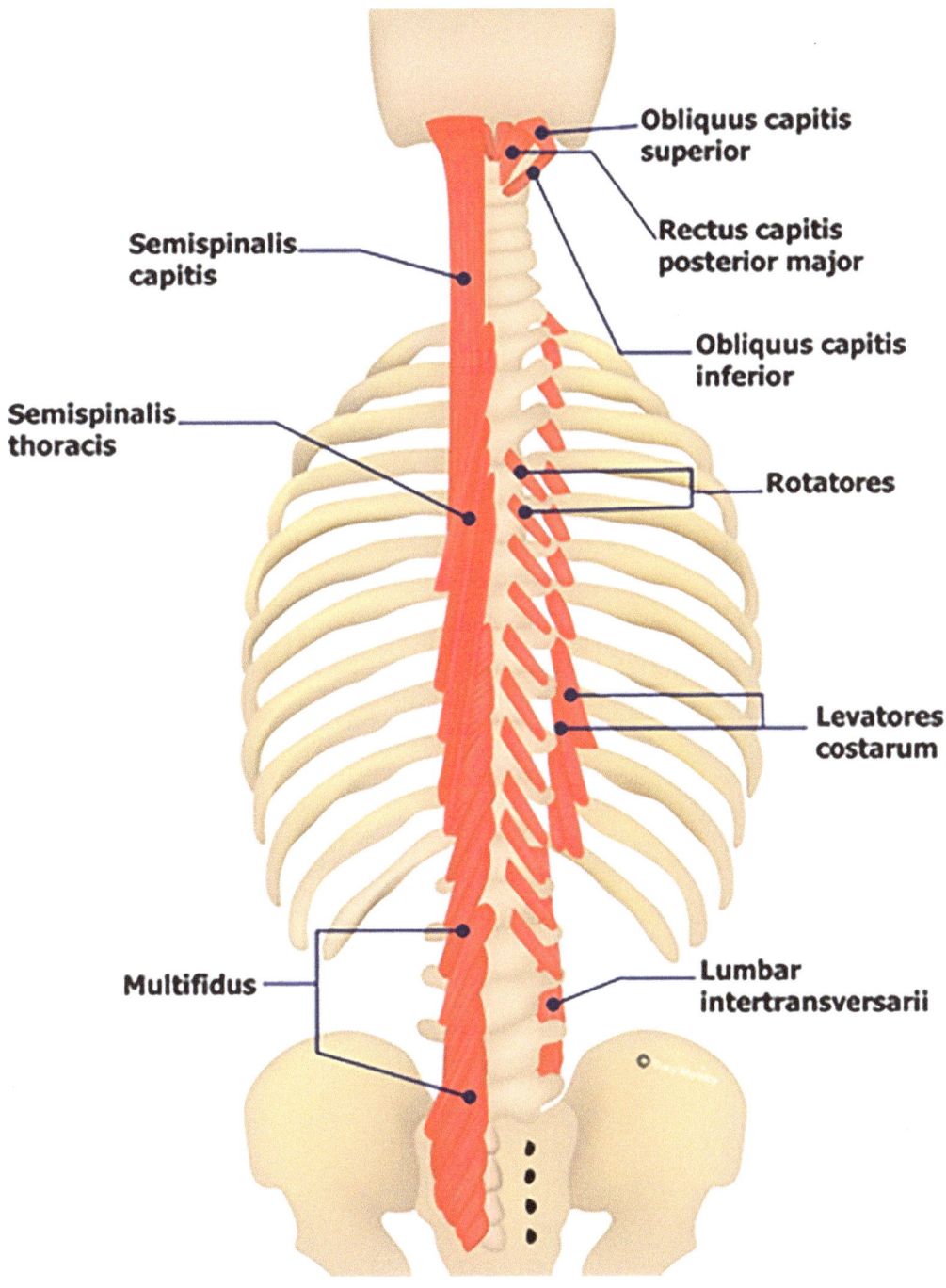

Obliquus capitis superior

Rectus capitis posterior major

Obliquus capitis inferior

Semispinalis capitis

Semispinalis thoracis

Rotatores

Levatores costarum

Multifidus

Lumbar intertransversarii

In the illustration above, the right side shows sections only for learning purposes. They are not drawn to show their full attachments throughout the spine.

The **Transversospinalis group** consists of:

The **rotators**, **interspinales,** and intertransversarii.

These muscles are essential for providing proprioception feedback between the brain, the back and entire body.

Rotators – The job of these muscles is to extend the spine and aid rotation to the opposite side. They move with proprioception, bringing balance when the body is in movement. They are the deepest and most medial layer of spinal fascial. They extend the spine and rotation to the opposite side. This group of muscles has a lot to do with proprioception, especially the rotators and the interspinales. The interspinales have a lot to do with the feedback between the back and brain and from brain to back. They are the deepest, (deeper than the multifidus) and have the most medial layer of spinal fascia. Medial meaning: the closest to the middle of the body.

Interspinales – Segmental extension. This muscle brings a lot of proprioception for the back, balance and stability of spine and body in movement. Segmental extension of the spine means arching the back.

Intertransversarii – Small segmental motion and lateral flexion of the spine.

They are small muscles that are on both sides of the spine.

The Interspinales and Intertransversarii muscles move and stabilize the spine. They also play a large role in body awareness and proprioception.

Therefore, it is so important to strengthen the core and spine from the inside out. The body communicates for movement, which begins deep in the spine. Therefore, when I train clients to regain the ability and cognitive skills such as balance, spatial awareness, and proprioception, I begin with simple, but extremely effective exercises. I have them stand on balance discs, balance pads, and/or BOSU® balls, to rebuild these muscles and their natural communication to the brain and back.

Included in the previous illustration are these muscles:

Obliquus Capitis Superior, Rectus Capitis Posterior Major, Obliquus Capitis Inferior, and the Levatores Costarum. All these and the Multifidus are small muscles that run along the spine from the skull to the sacrum. They extend, abduct, adduct, and rotate the spine.

These small but powerful spine muscles must be strong for the spine to move safely without injury and to have a truly strong core.

Quadratus Lumborum

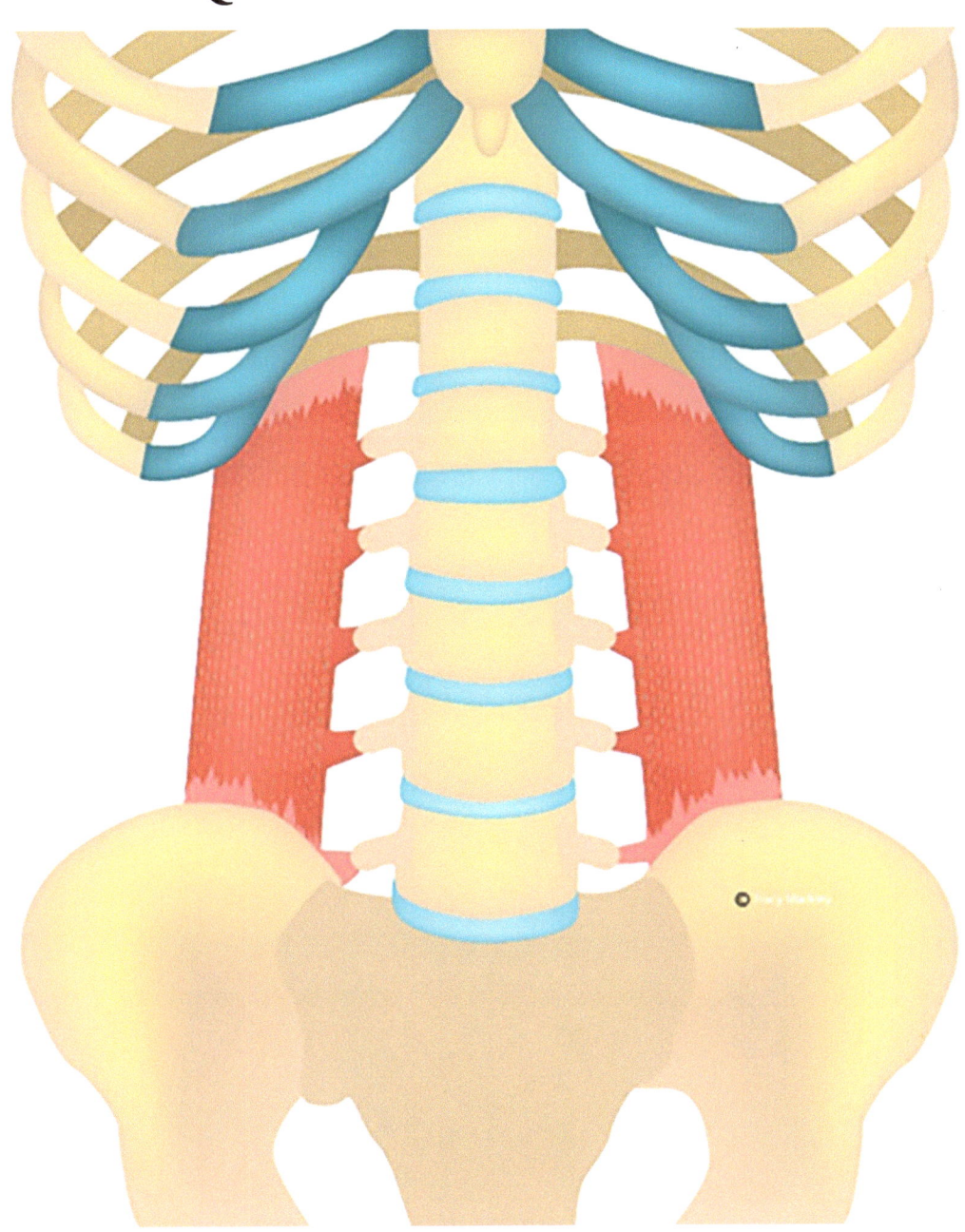

The quadratus lumborum (as you can see in the illustration above) is attached from the lumbar vertebrae and rib 12 to the crest of the ilium. It stabilizes the pelvis (hip girdle) in walking and laterally flexes the spine. It performs lateral flexion like you saw in the seven (7) positional movements of the spine chapter. It has three layers of fibers that move in three different directions. The quadratus lumborum can cause a lot of pain if having issues or a bad injury. When this muscle is only activated (or in spasticity) on one side, the trunk is bent towards that direction.

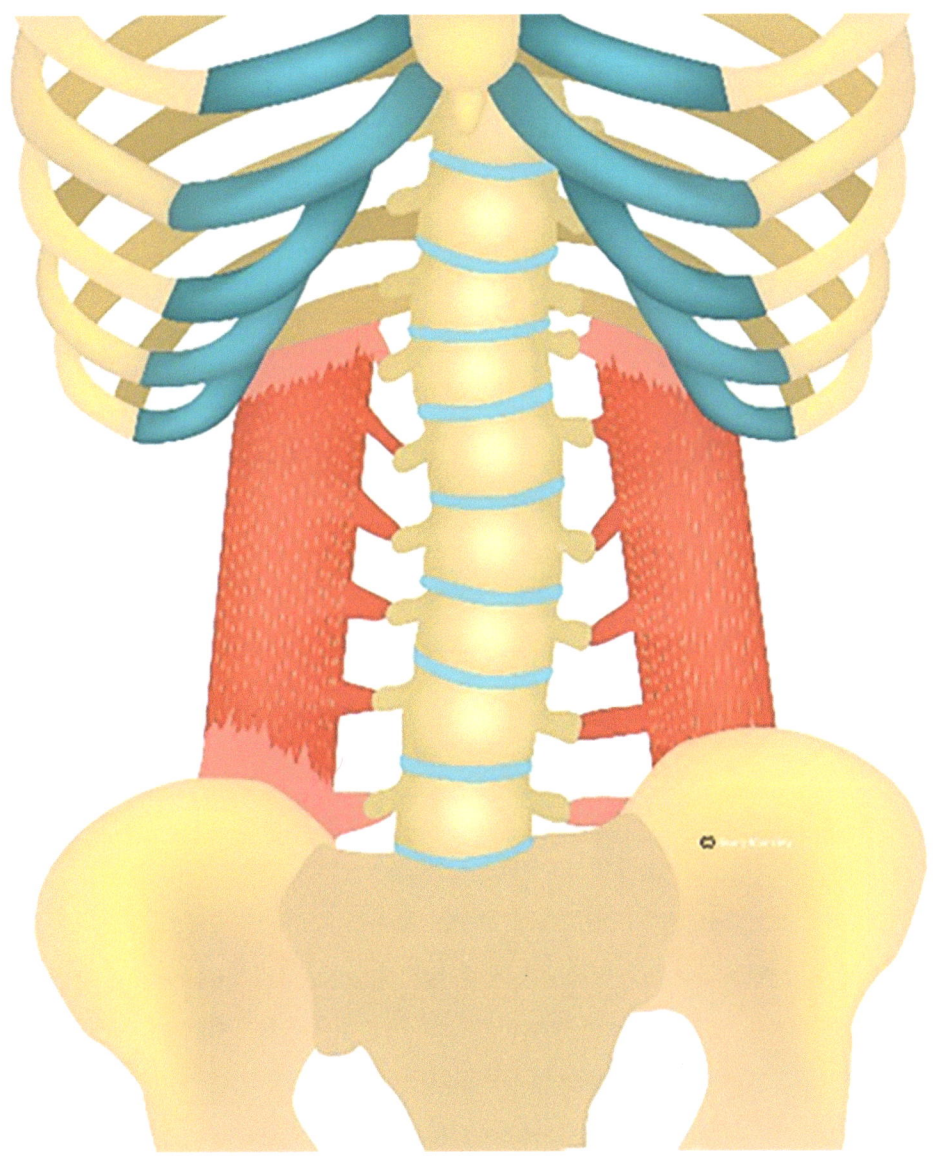

This illustration of the **Quadratus Lumborum** (QT) shows how when one side of the QT is shorter than the other side, it can hike up the pelvis/hips. This will affect the whole body. When someone sits with their hips off to one side, this is what the psoas and other smaller and larger spine muscles are doing as well. They are developing an imbalance on both sides of the spine, which leads to malfunction in many movements. Remember when the body is in a proper position, all the systems in the body work better.

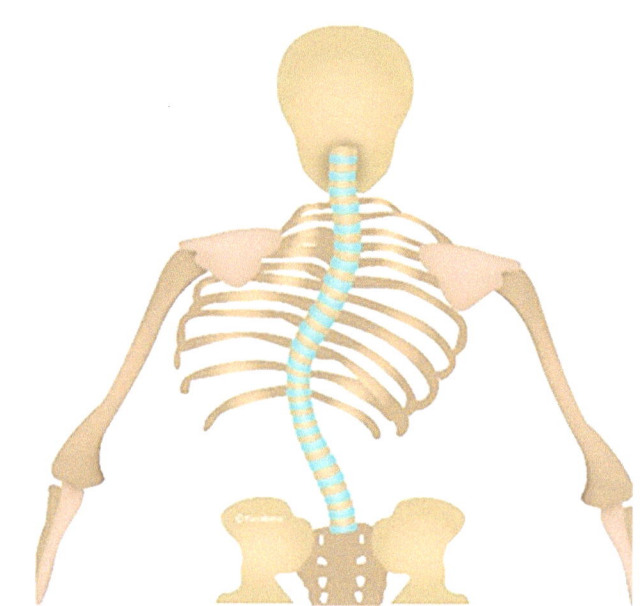

With scoliosis, this sort of muscle imbalance is going on. Some may have scoliosis due to poor posture, stroke, injury, playing sports, and other reasons that can be corrected by careful and conscious exercises, stretches, and therapy. Others may have been born with it or developed it by life and disease, and some have a very extreme case. You can see in the second illustration the severity and the many muscles that would be out of balance and affected by the spinal curve.

For example, if someone is trying to learn to walk again and they spend much time sitting with the muscles in this position, when they try to stand or walk, they will not have the strength, balance, and muscle connection to regain the skill at their best or often not at all.

These illustrations are also another visual to show the power of the spine muscles.

Erector Spinae

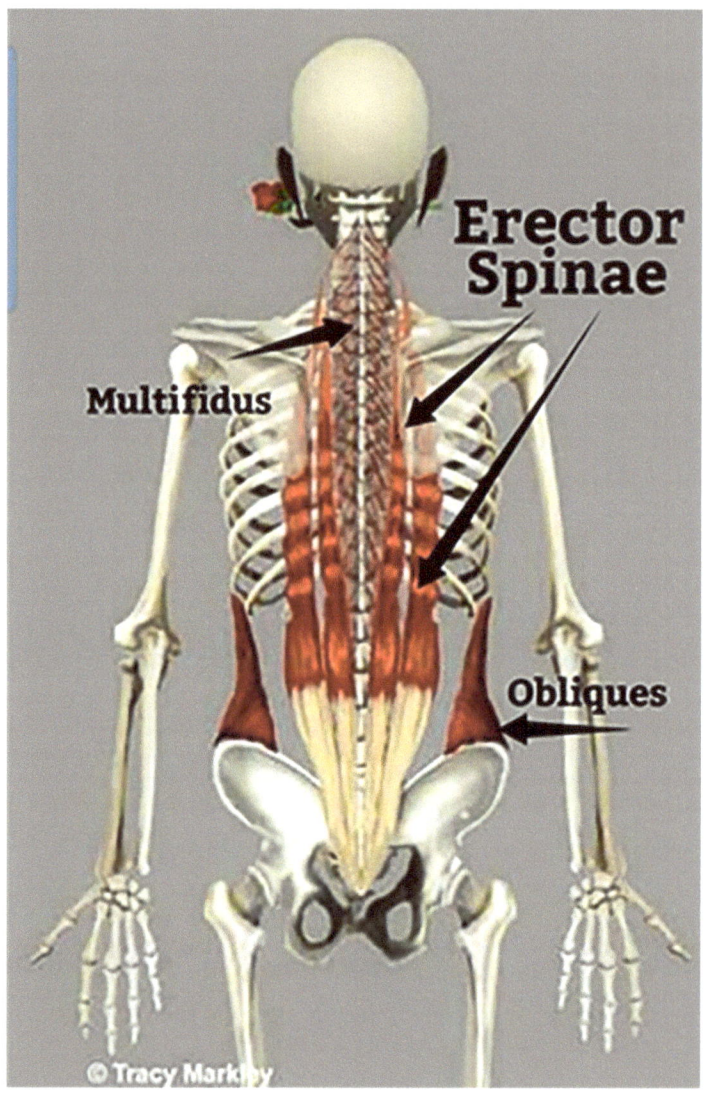

FYI - @motivate_healthyfit is my Instagram account name.

The Erector Spinae muscles consist of the Longissimus, Iliocostalis, and Spinalis. They each run parallel on the outer side of the vertebrae on both sides of the spine. They extend from the lower part of the skull to the pelvis. These muscles straighten the back and help provide some stabilization for side-to-side rotation. Injury to these muscles can cause back spasms and pain.

In this illustration, you see the diaphragm and the psoas muscle and the pelvic floor. I share this to give another visual of how the psoas (a spine muscle) connects to both the femurs (leg bone) and its close connection with the diaphragm.

Latissimus Dorsi and Thoracolumbar Fascia

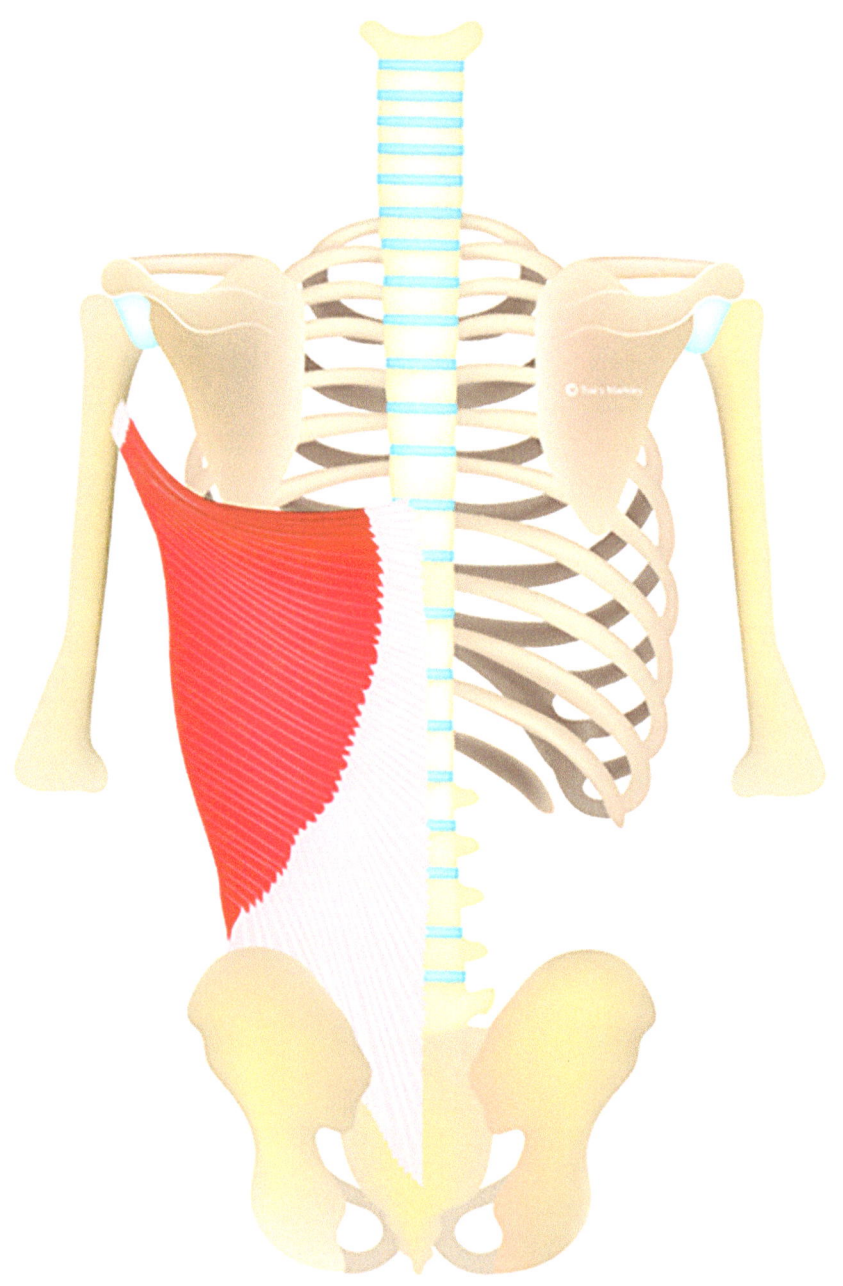

The **Latissimus Dorsi** attaches at the hip and back and into the **thoracolumbar fascia** to the humerus (the upper arm bone). The **thoracolumbar fascia** supports the back muscles and helps them achieve the ability to move the body. It is made up of strong fibers and helps channel forces of movement, as the back muscles contract and relax. The nerves to these muscles also cross through this fascia. This fascia goes deep to the spine and is made of three layers. It is essential for contralateral motions like walking. It works with the latissimus dorsi (lats) to coil the core of the body.

When the **thoracolumbar fascia** is supported, it allows all the muscles that connect to it to function better. These muscles include the gluteus maximus, latissimus dorsi, trapezius, erector spine, quadratus lumborum, psoas, transverse, and internal obliques. It helps bridge the muscles of the back to the muscles of the abdominal wall. This fascia helps integrate the movements of the upper body with the lower body.

We also have a posterior Oblique Subsystem (which is not the exact opposite of the oblique abdominal muscles despite the similar name). This system consists of:

- Latissimus Dorsi Muscle

- Thoracolumbar Fascia (not a muscle)

- Contralateral Gluteus Maximus Muscle (Some also consider the Gluteus Medius a part as well.)

By now, you should have a better understanding of the great importance of the spine, back, core, and how all the muscles work together as a team and individually to support and move the whole body.

I greatly believe in the Spinal Engine Theory by Serge Gracovetsky. It links the spinal engine to the walking gait and power behind running speeds. The motivational speaker Nick Vujucic was born with no limbs. When he moves, swims, and walks, it shows just how truly powerful the spine and core are.

EXTRA IMPORTANT NOTE:

What is Fascia? Fascia is a tough connective tissue that connects and intertwines through the whole body. It surrounds every muscle, muscle fibers, spindles, and continues through attaching with tendons.

Fascia is about 70% water. Dehydration and staying slightly dehydrated by not drinking enough water will cause negative fascial issues throughout the body. Stay hydrated for your brain, muscles, organs, and fascia.

If you did not know:

Ligaments attach bone to bone. Tendons attach muscle to bone.

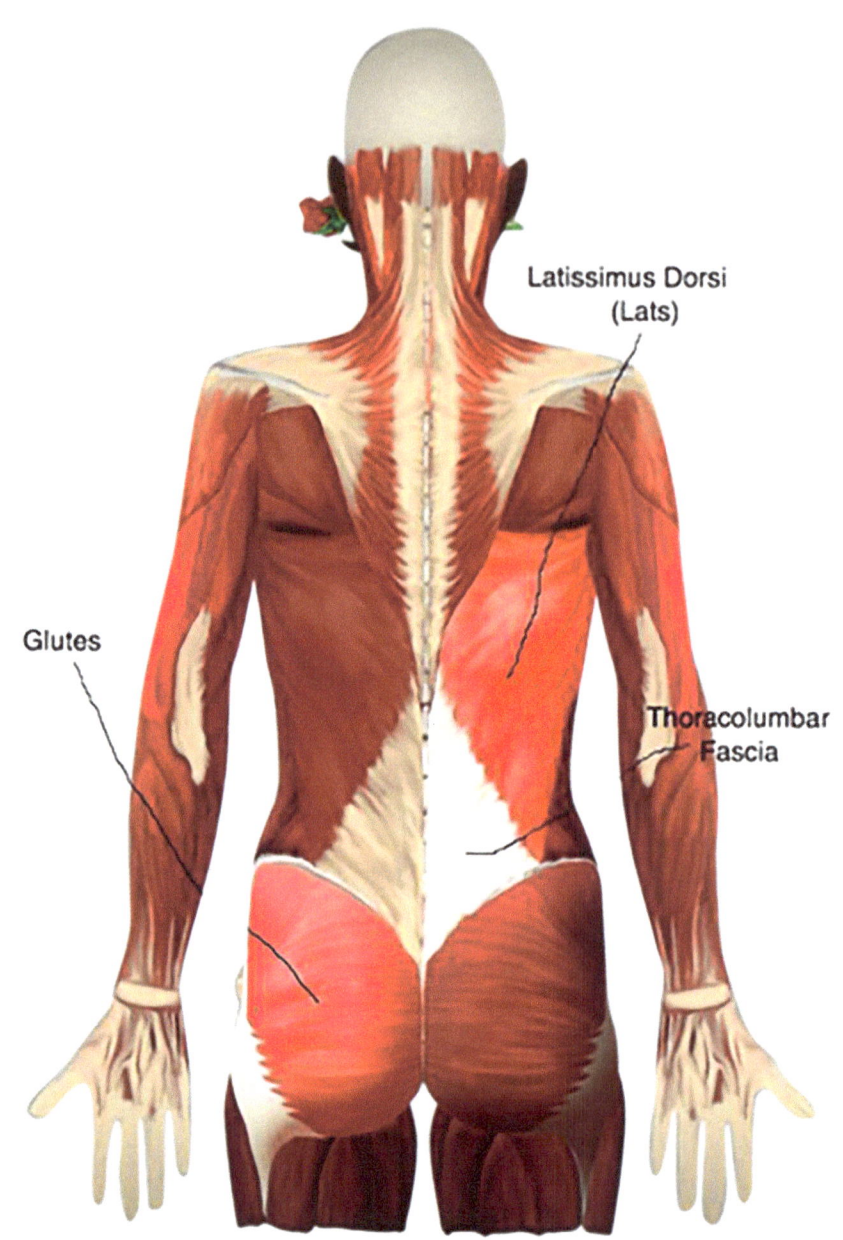

An extra image to see how the muscle fibers of the Latissimus Dorsi and the Glutes flow through and with the Thoracolumbar Fascia.

Trapezius Muscle and other muscles

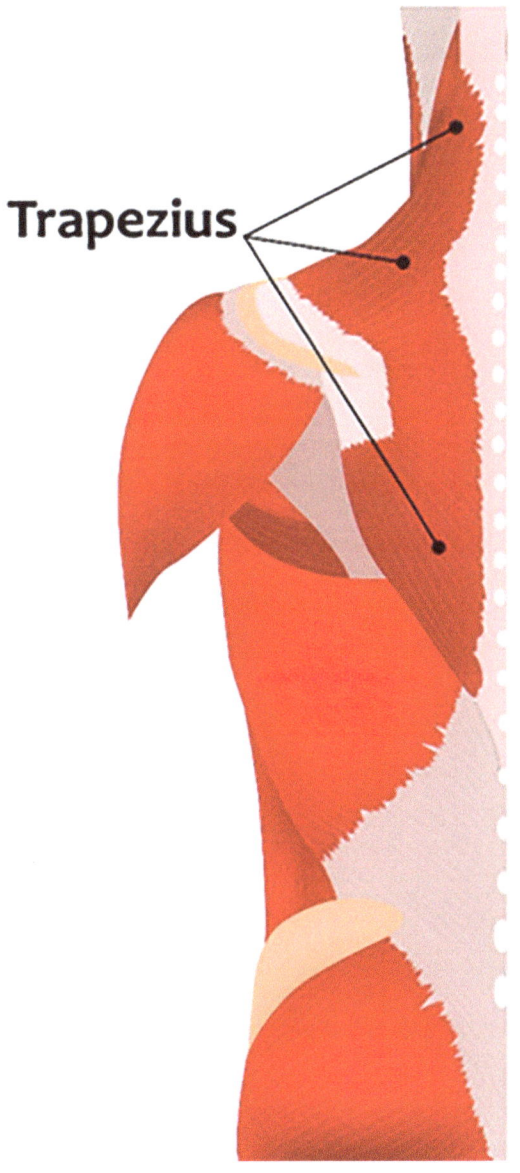

The **Trapezius** muscle is in three sections. The superior, medial, and inferior. Superior meaning above. Medial meaning middle. Inferior meaning lower.

The **Superior Trapezius** attaches to the scapula, to the skull, and to the vertebrae. It abducts the scapula.

The **Medial Trapezius** attaches horizontally from the scapula to the vertebrae. It abducts and rotates the scapula inward.

The **Inferior Trapezius** attaches to the scapula and to the vertebrae below. It abducts and rotates the scapula inward.

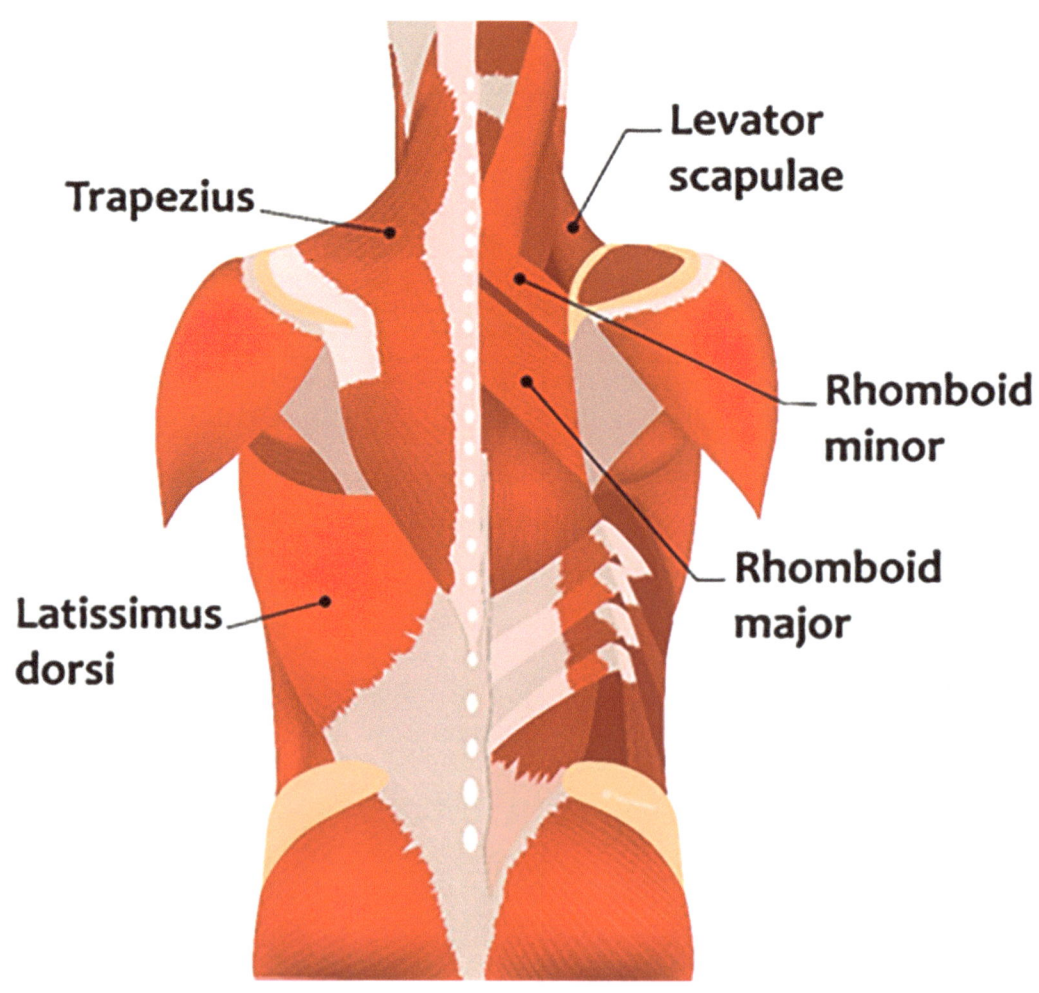

Levator Scapulae

The Levator Scapulae attaches at the scapula and the cervical vertebrae above. It abducts and adducts the spine. Levator means elevator.

We also have the **Sternocleidomastoid** muscle.

Not shown in the illustration.

The **Sternocleidomastoid** attaches at the sternum, clavicle, and mastoid process.

It flexes, abducts, adducts, and rotates the spine.

There are other small muscles around the neck and upper shoulder area that are not mentioned in this book, but they each have their own individual roles in movements of the upper spine.

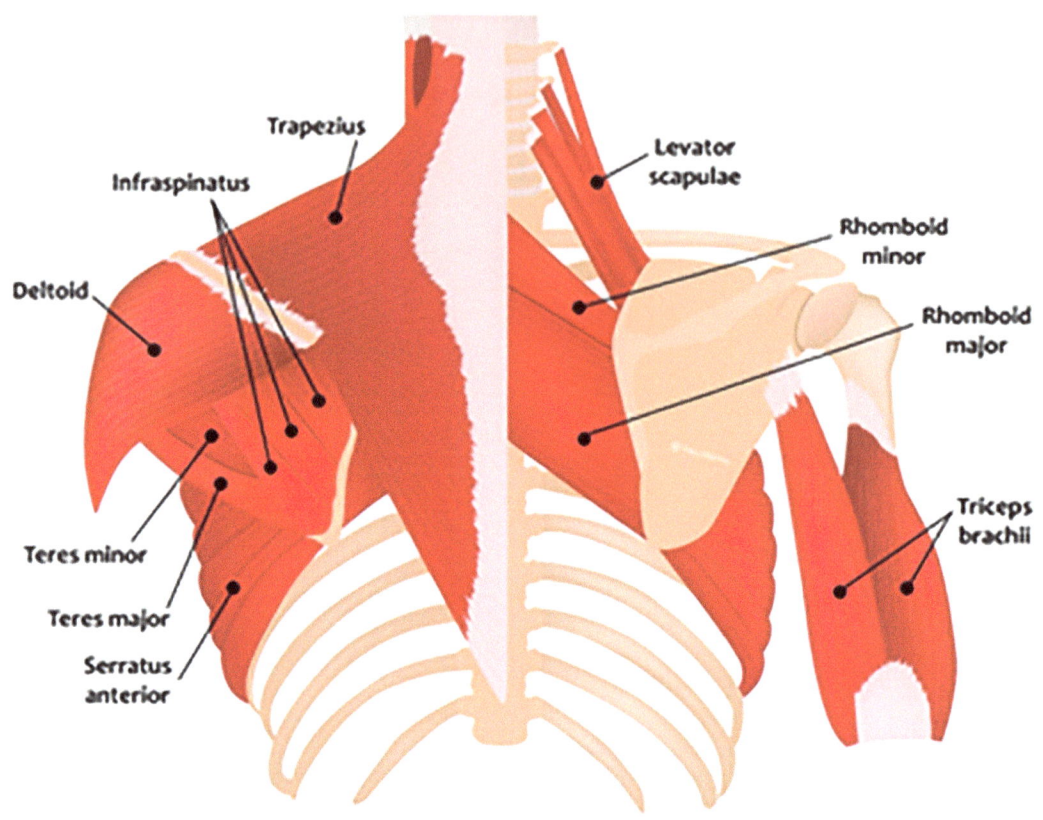

Most of the muscles above have already been mentioned except the Teres Major and the Serratus Anterior.

Teres Major Muscle attaches to the scapula and the humerus. It assists in the extension and medial rotation of the humerus.

Teres Minor Muscle is one of the rotator cuff muscles mentioned later in the book. It attaches to the scapula and the humerus. It laterally rotates the arm and stabilizes the humerus.

Serratus Anterior Muscle is attached at the scapula and to ribs 1 through 9. It rotates scapula outward.

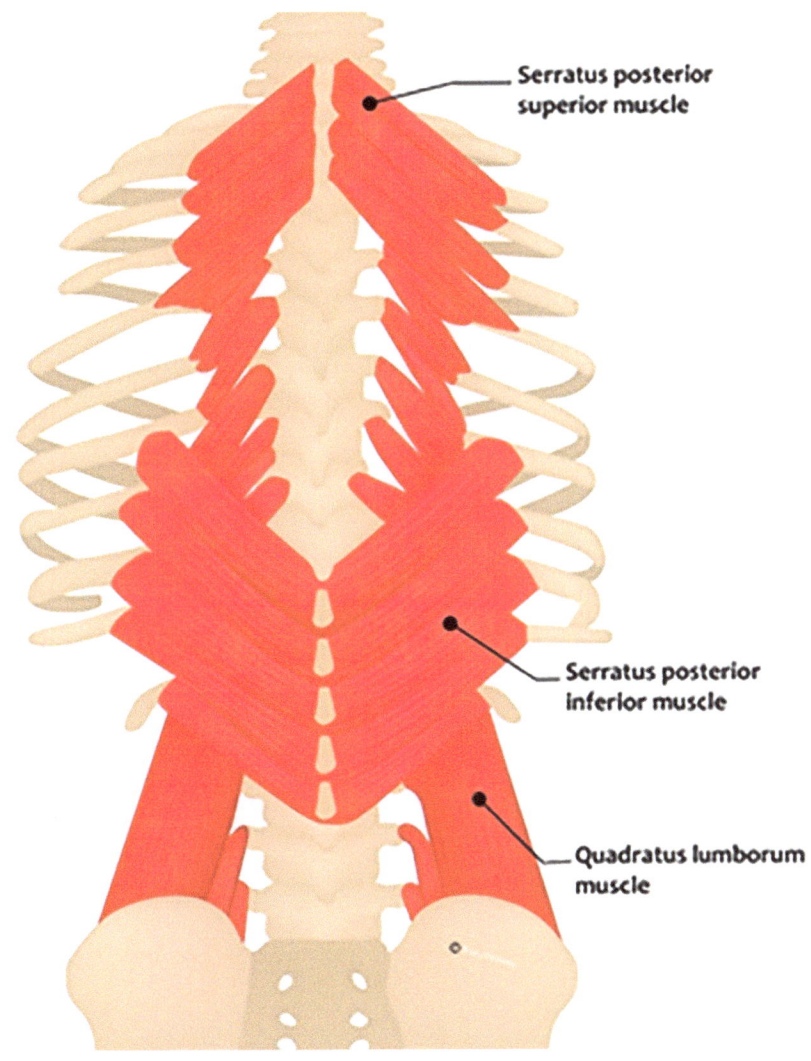

I previously shared the **Serratus Anterior** in another illustration. I did not mention that many body builders like to get a nice cut of definition in that muscle.

You also have a **Serratus Posterior Superior** and a **Serratus Posterior Inferior** muscles.

The **Serratus Posterior Superior** attaches at C7 (7th Cervical vertebrae) through T3 (3rd Thoracic vertebrae) and to the 2nd through 5th ribs. It elevates (abducts) the ribs during inhalation.

The **Serratus Posterior Inferior** attaches at T11 (11th Thoracic vertebrae) through L2 (2nd Lumbar vertebrae). It adducts the ribs during exhalation and prevents the ribs from pulling through the diaphragm.

Often, people keep their ribs elevated in an attempt to achieve good posture. When in fact, this can cause low back pain.

The Serratus Posterior Inferior attaches to lumbar vertebrae and the four ribs above. This is an important thing to remember, so you can have proper posture whether you are standing around, lifting, or exercising. Intense Certified Pilates instructors teach this. I love Pilates' and incorporating Joseph Pilates teachings with all exercise modalities.

An important thing to know:

The **transverse abdominal muscle**, the **multifidus muscle, diaphragm,** and the **pelvic floor muscles** are all on the same neuromuscular loop. This means it is best if all these muscles are functioning properly; each needs to perform its job individually <u>and</u> as a team. If the transverse muscle is weak, the pelvic floor, the multifidus and the diaphragm cannot gain proper strength to perform their jobs in a healthy, functioning body.

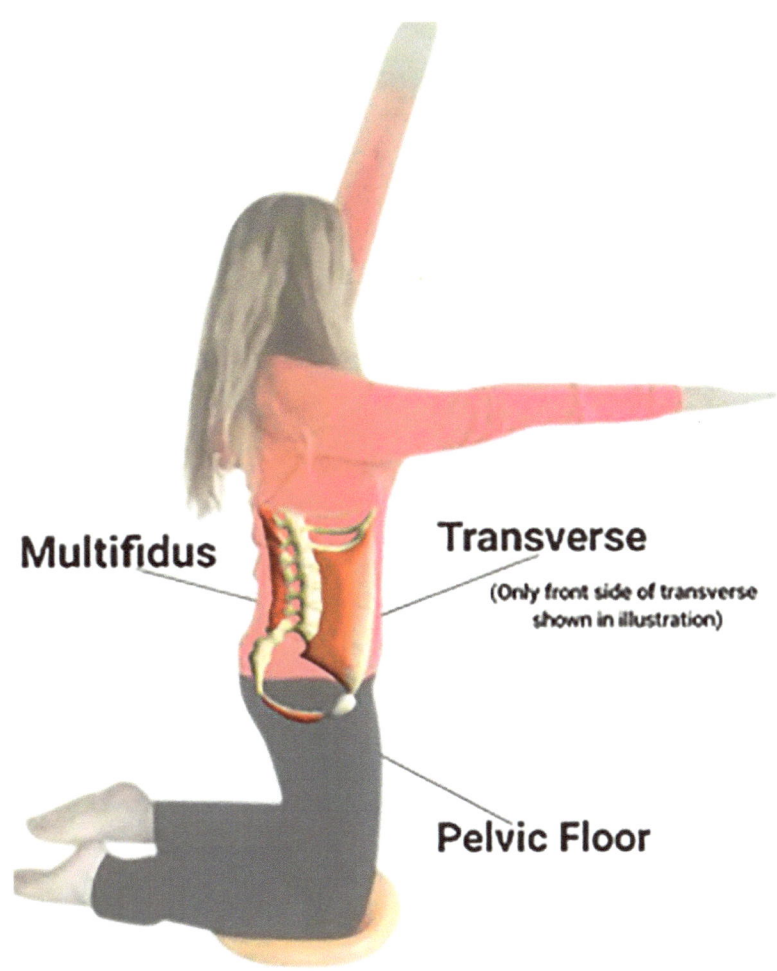

Multifidus

Transverse

(Only front side of transverse shown in illustration)

Pelvic Floor

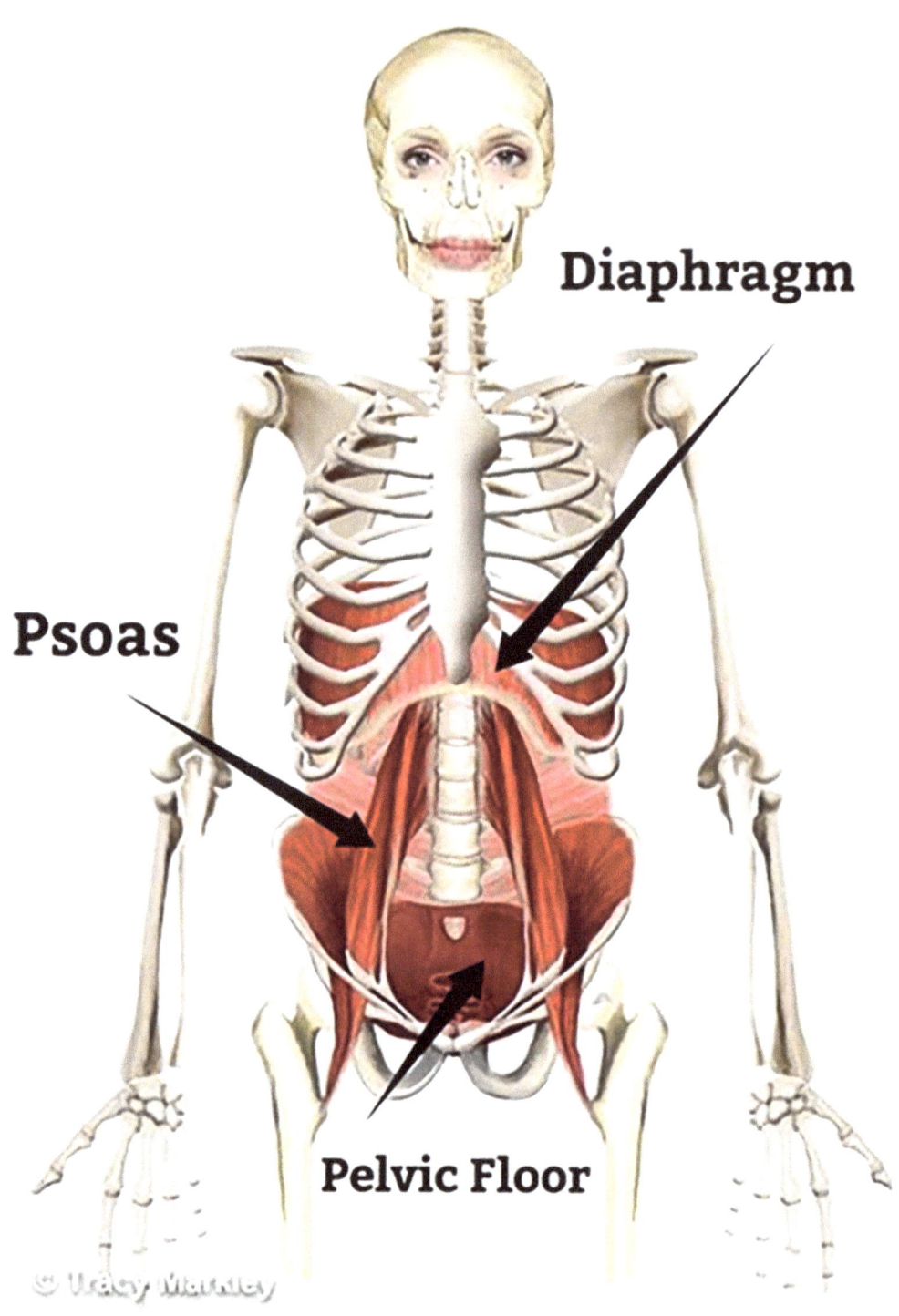

Diaphragm

Psoas

Pelvic Floor

© Tracy Markley

CHAPTER 5

ABDOMINAL MUSCLES

Supporting, Protecting, and Helping to Assist in

Spinal Movement

Rectus Abdominus

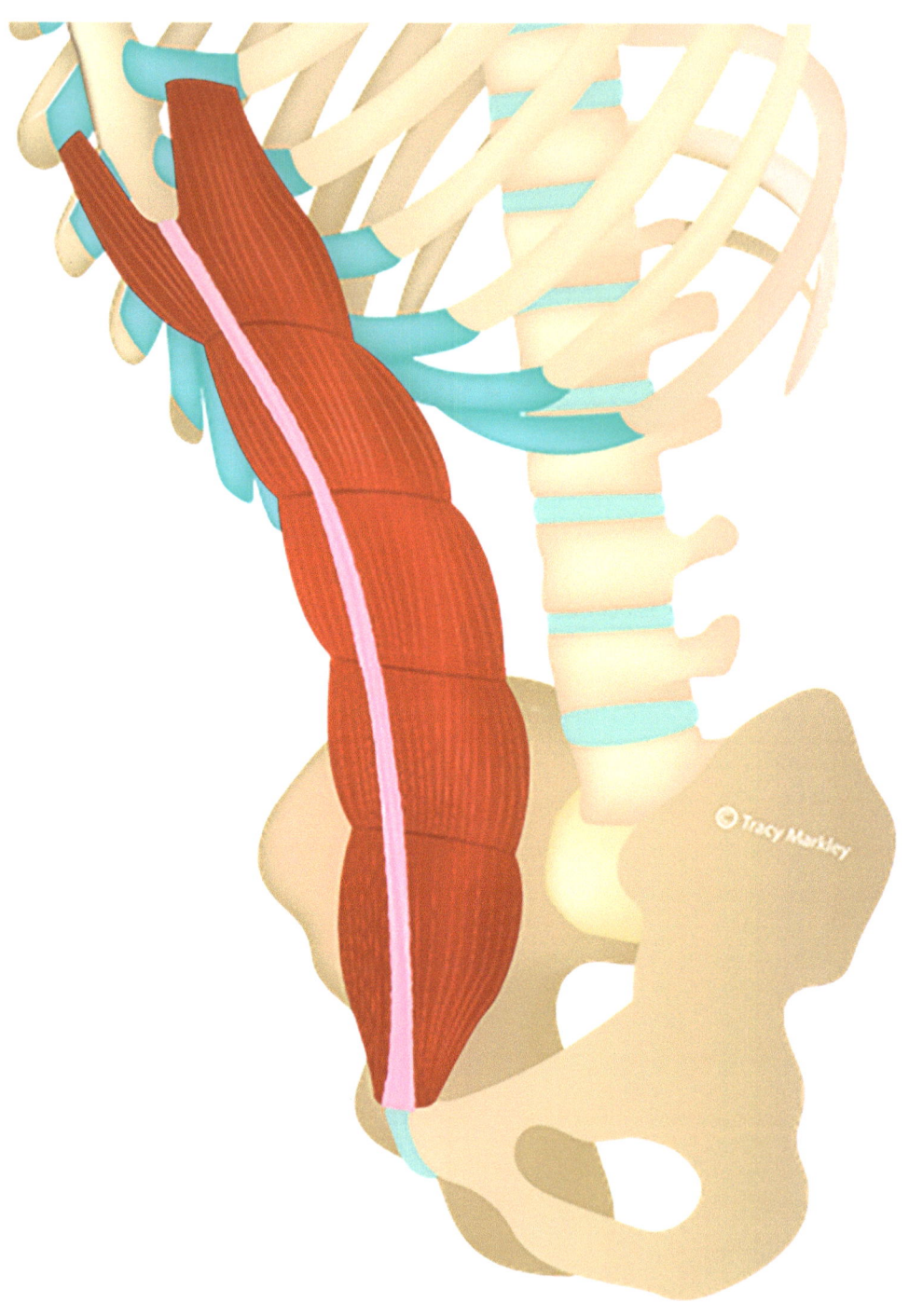

The **rectus abdominus** is the abdominal muscle closest to the surface. This is the muscle that creates the "six-pack" appearance. It attaches at the front of the ribs 5 through 7 and to the pubis. It flexes and adducts the spine and enables the tilt of the pelvis and the curvature of the low spine. The rectus abdominus also adducts the ribs causing exhalation. Often, when people just do abdominal crunches and no real functional training of the abs and core, this muscle can get tight, adding or causing back pain.

Internal Oblique Muscles

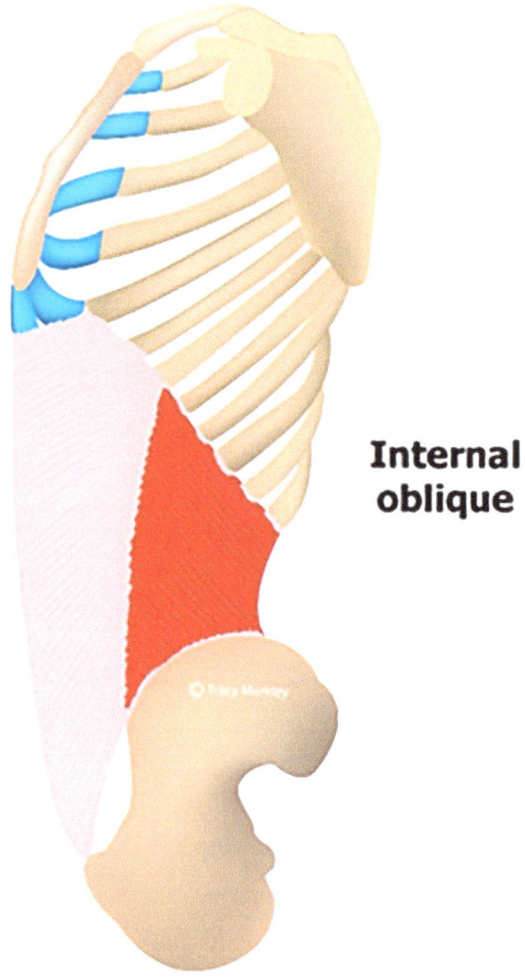

Internal oblique

The word "oblique," according to the Oxford Dictionary, means neither parallel nor a right angle to a line, but slanting or an angle. Both the Internal and External Oblique muscle fibers run on an angle.

The **Internal Oblique** is on the lateral (side) aspect of the trunk. It attaches at ribs 10 through 12 and to the crest of the ilium (pelvic bone). It adducts the ribs, causing exhalation. It also flexes, abducts, and adducts and rotates the spine.

External Oblique Muscles

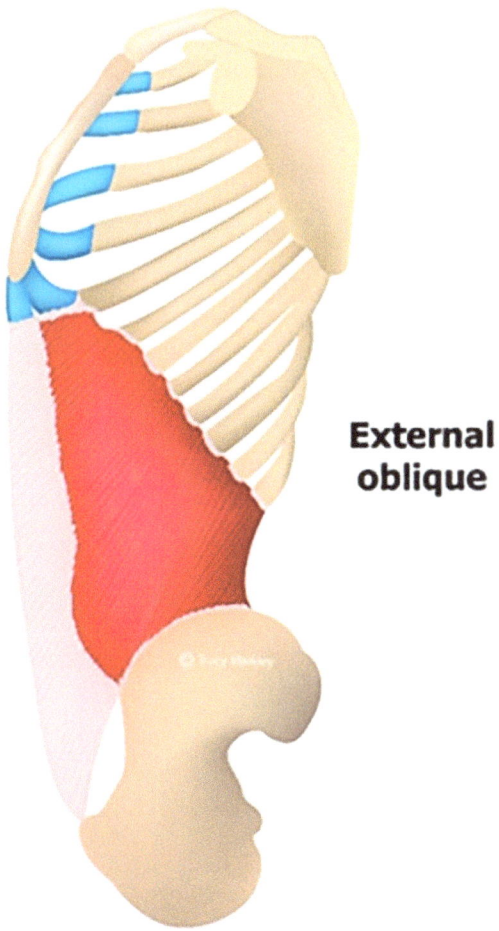

External oblique

The **External Oblique** attaches from rib 5 through 12 and to the crest of the ilium. It adducts the ribs causing exhalation and flexes and adducts and rotates the spine.

If the deep spinal muscles that you read about earlier in this book are weak and not performing their job properly, these outer muscles will pull harder on the spine leading to injury and malfunction. It is very important to strengthen the body from the inside out like a baby develops. This is a key to balance, spine and back care, proprioception, stabilization, and protection of the spine. It is also the key to building all the spine and core muscles to their best strength, so all the muscles can focus on only the job they were made to do. This also leaves the body less fatigued.

Transverse Abdominal Muscle

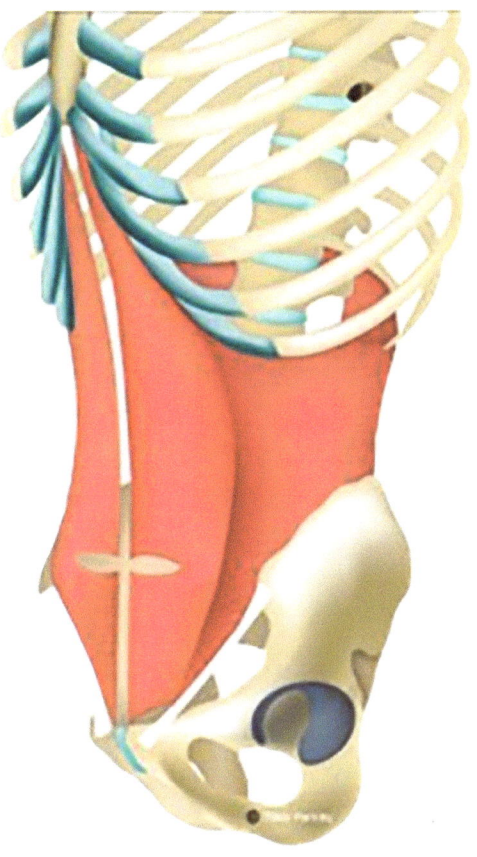

The **transverse muscle** is the deepest of the abdominal muscles. This is not a spine or back muscle, but without this muscle being strong, the **multifidus spine muscle** cannot be strong. The **transverse muscle's** critical function is to stabilize the lower back and pelvis before movement. It is the deepest abdominal muscle, wrapping around the body to act like a corset. It helps stabilize the hips and pelvic. When engaged, it also pulls the belly in and provides support to the **thoracolumbar fascia.** The transverse is also the stabilizer of the shoulder girdle, the head, neck, pelvis, and lower extremities.

For those who are trying to correct posture or are in rehabilitation to learn to stand and walk again or someone who has rounded shoulders and poor posture, it is essential to strengthen this muscle. It must be strengthened to help the other stabilizing muscles hold the body strongly upright and achieve a posture in which the shoulders are stacked over the hips. If our head is upright and balanced over the shoulders, we have better balance. The stability in the pelvis and hips is necessary, so that the lower limbs and joints can gain strength, function in alignment, and perform properly for safe movements.

Before we move forward to another muscle, I hope it is becoming clearer to you just how muscles work together to help other muscles in the body perform their jobs.

The **pelvic floor** muscles work as stabilizers of the abdominal and pelvic organs. The pelvic floor muscles and the gluteus (buttock) muscles are made to work and move in opposite directions. One must be able to engage the pelvic floor without engaging the gluteus muscles in order to obtain optimal core strength. These two muscles must be separated in the brain and nervous system for overall whole-body functioning. This plays a role in preventing back issues, and I don't want to build back issues in any client. The transverse muscle must be strong for the pelvic floor to become strong and function properly, since they are on the same neuromuscular loop.

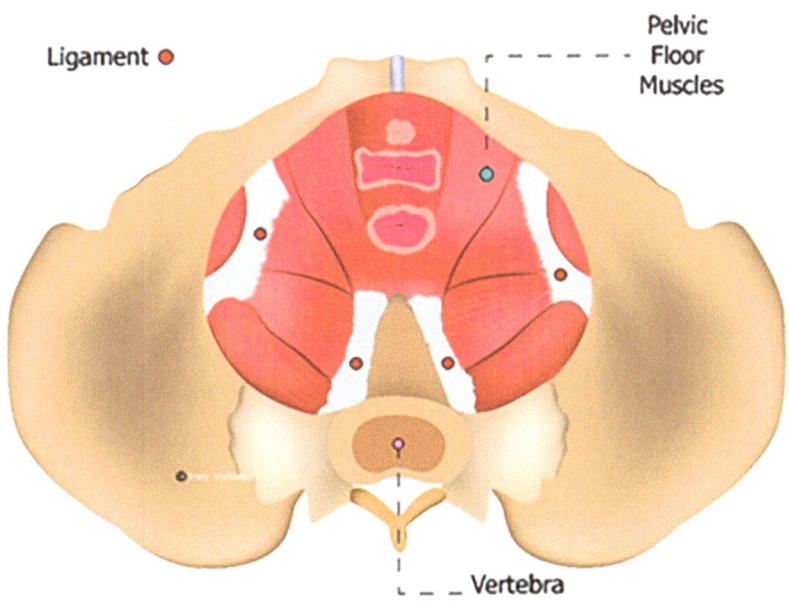

The **pelvic floor** works close to the diaphragm as well. If you sit or stand in good alignment and focus on engaging the pelvic floor, you can feel that the diaphragm pulls slightly towards the pelvic floor as the pelvic floor lifts slightly towards the diaphragm. There is a difference between doing a Kegel and engaging the pelvic floor. It is also important to be able to engage the pelvic floor without engaging the buttocks (glutes) for the inner unit and stabilizing system in the body to work efficiently.

The Glutes

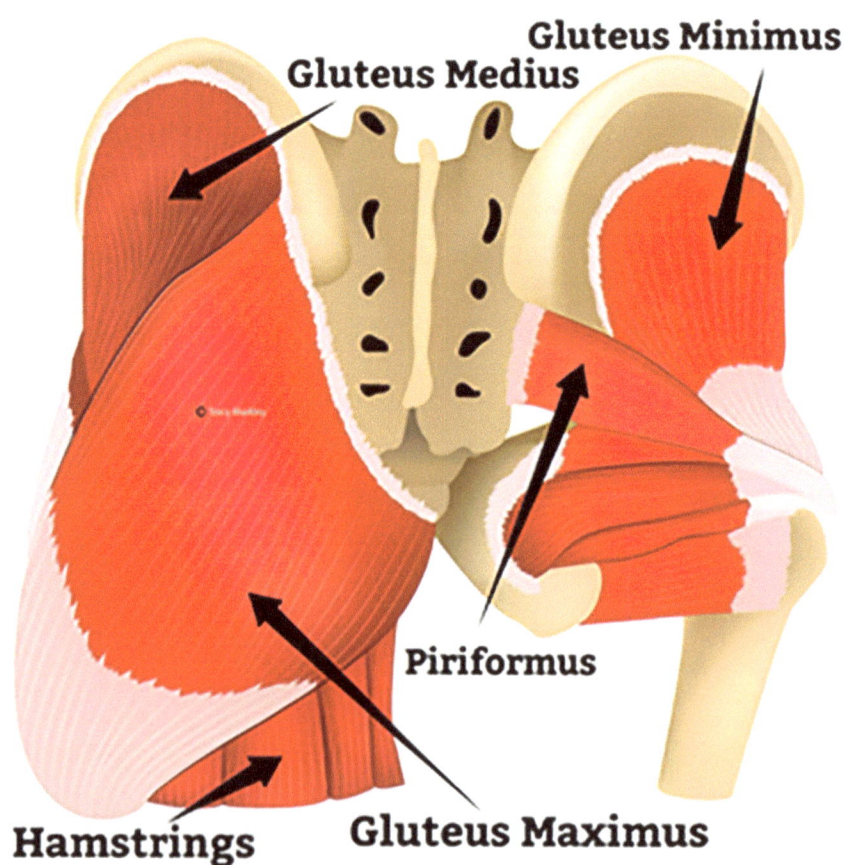

In this illustration, you will see the large glute muscles and the smaller muscles that are underneath. The large glute muscles extend the femur, which is the back swing of the leg in walking. It also rotates the femur outward. The smaller group of muscles work together to rotate the femur outward. The femur is the large upper thigh bone.

We have a gluteus maximus, medius, and minimus. The gluteus maximus extends and rotates the femur outward, while the gluteus medius and minimus abducts and rotates the femur inward.

If the spine and back muscles are weak and there is poor posture, the hips and pelvic will not be strong and stable enough to allow the glute muscles and other muscles like the piriformis and the other hip rotator muscles you see in this illustration to work properly. This leaves the spine and back muscles to try to assist in these muscles' jobs, leaving the body trying to function and moving out of balance causing pain, weakness, and injury in the back as well as hips, knees, and ankles. Posture is essential.

NOTES

CHAPTER 6

THE SCIATIC NERVE: THE GOOD AND THE UGLY

As trainers and therapists, when we hear "sciatic nerve," we instantly think of pain.

Although the sciatic nerve is said to be the largest single nerve in the body, it is made up of five nerves. It is found on the right and left side of the lower spine by the fourth and fifth lumbar nerves and the first three nerves in the sacral spine. At the largest part of the nerve, it is as big as a male thumb. The five nerves gather together on the front of the piriformis muscles and become one large nerve known as the sciatic nerve.

This nerve supplies sensation and strength to the leg and the reflexes of the leg. It connects the spinal cord with the outside of the thigh, the hamstring muscles, and the muscles of the lower leg and feet. It provides motor and sensory functions to regions of the leg and foot. When the sciatic nerve is impaired, it can lead to muscle weakness and/or numbness and tingling in the leg, ankle, foot, and toes. The sciatic nerve and its nerve branches enable movement and feeling in the thigh, knee, calf, ankle, foot, and toes.

This nerve exits the spinal cord between the 4th and 5th lumbar vertebrae, travels down both sides of the spine, and then through to the Piriformis muscles.

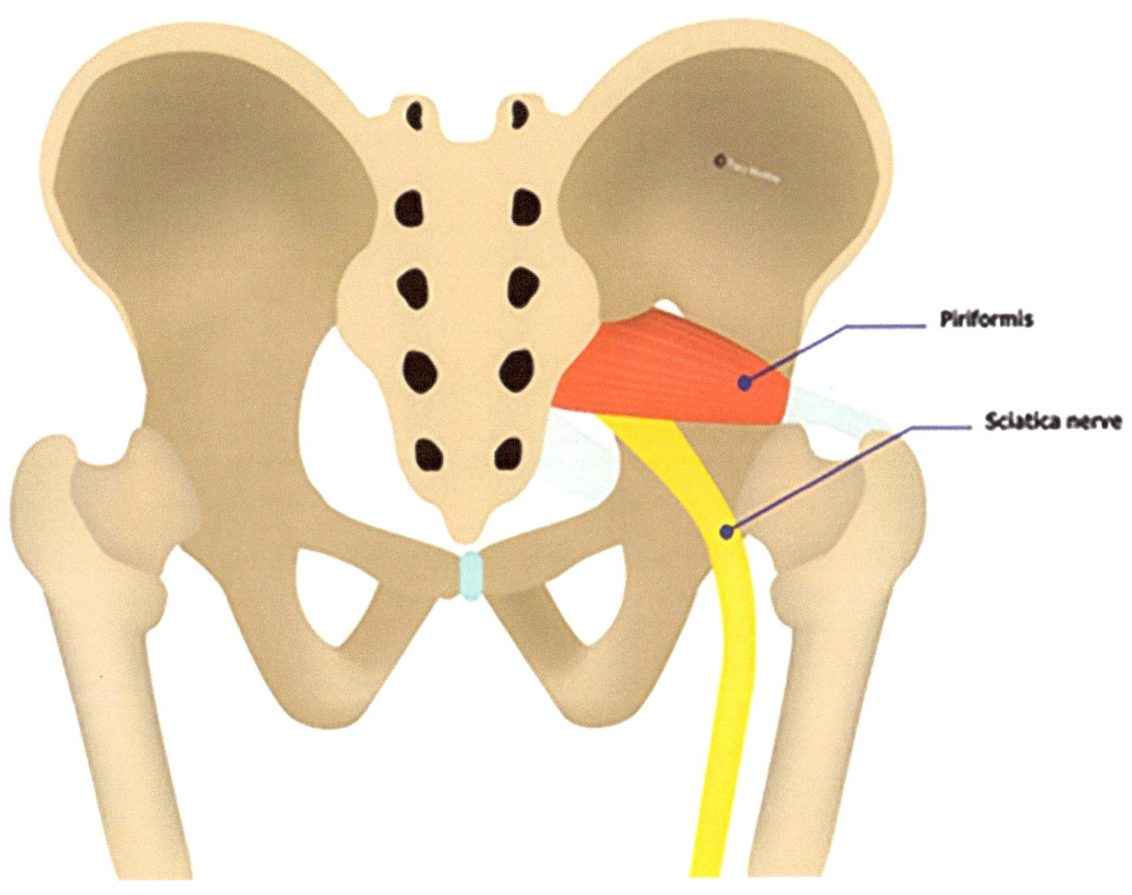

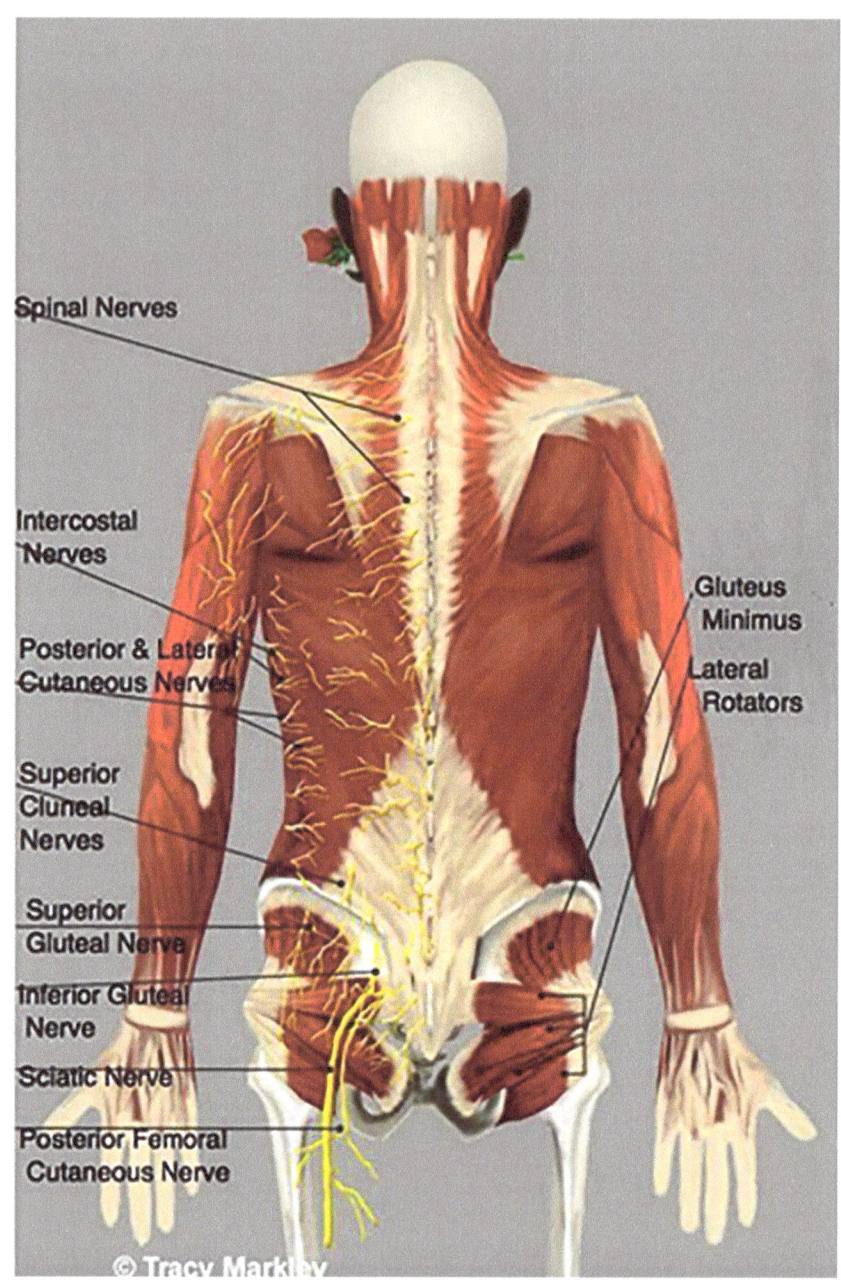

This illustration is an example of some of the nerves that cross through and with the back muscles and fascia.

Chapter 7

Other Muscles in the Body and How the Spine Affects Them And Vice Versa

The Rhomboids

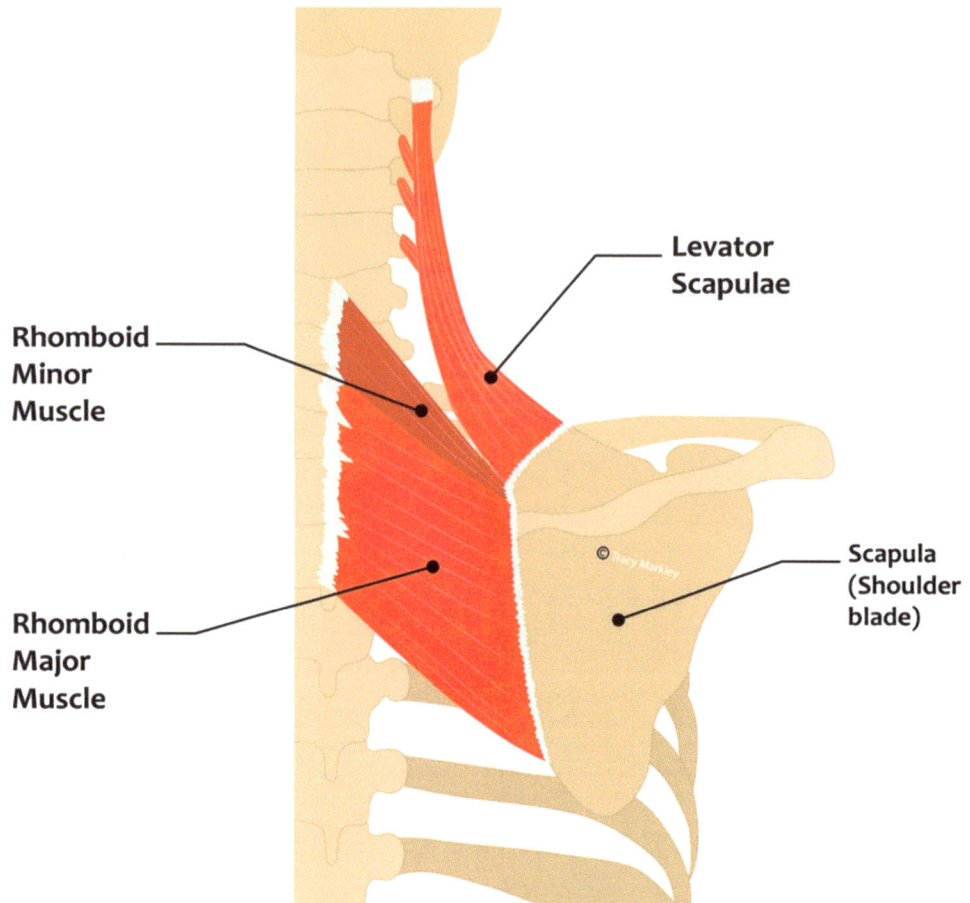

Rhomboid Major attaches at the scapula and the spine at the cervical vertebra (neck). It rotates inward and adducts the scapula.

Rhomboid Minor attaches scapula and the spine. It rotates inward and adducts the scapula.

The Rotator Cuff Muscles

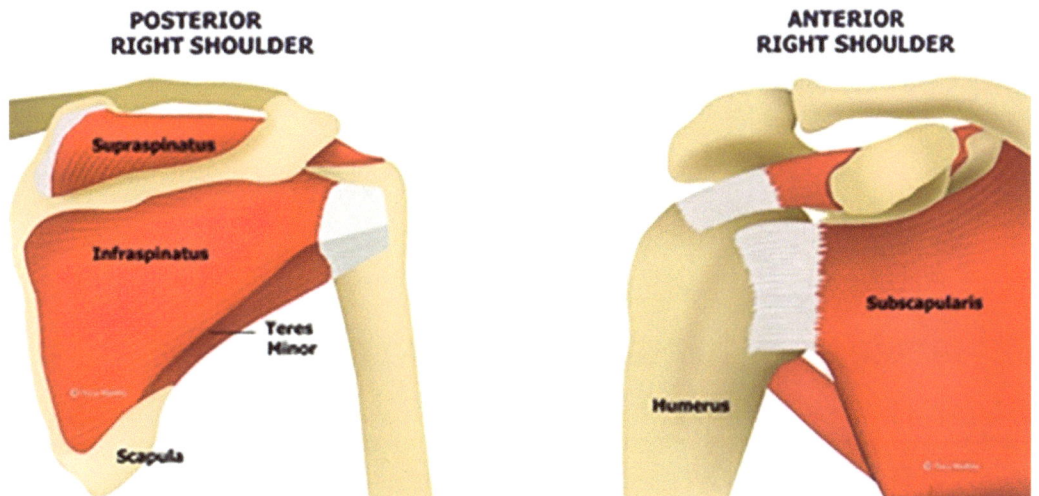

There are four muscles that make up what is known as the "rotator cuff."

These four muscles work together as a team to hold the shoulder girdle properly in place, so that the shoulder joint can move freely and safely. These four muscles are the **Supraspinatus**, **Infraspinatus**, **Teres Minor,** and **Subscapularis**. As they work as a team, they also have their own movements that they perform on their own. Poor posture and using the shoulder joint in poor form in everyday activities including exercising in all the different modalities will create an injury. It is common to hear a client say, they have a "rotator cuff injury" and not know which muscle or ligament it is. Many just assume it is a cuff and don't understand that there are these four muscles creating the so-called cuff.

As a trainer, it is sometimes difficult to determine what is causing a specific injury. If the client has poor posture such as rounded shoulders, when they do rehab exercise, he/she will not heal correctly. Good posture is essential.

When someone continually has their shoulders raised up into their ears, this puts the shoulder girdle and joint in a poor functioning movement, leading to injuries. It puts a pull on the fascia that goes through the body and spine. This leads to more back, hip, and pelvic pain in many people.

The stroke survivors I work with often have a partial or full shoulder dislocation. When it is put back in place and they keep their shoulder down, meaning they stop flexing the muscles that raise up the shoulders to the ears, the shoulder can then heal and get back in its proper position. It also helps relieve hip pain and tightness.

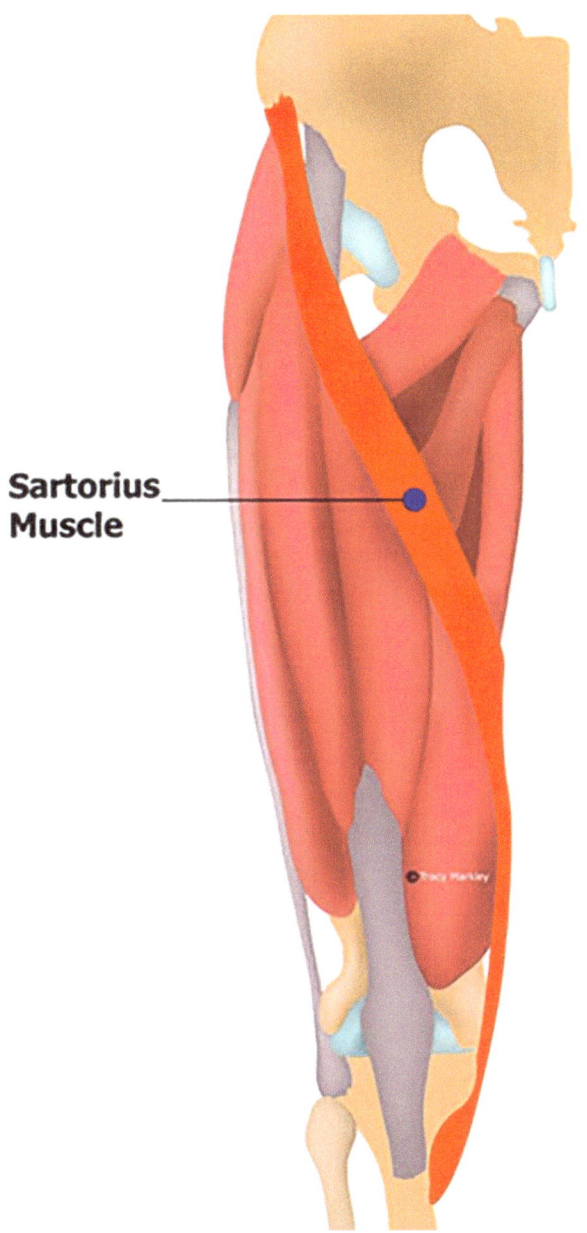

Highlighted here are the Sartorius muscle, the quadriceps, and others. They are the muscles of the front of the thigh.

The sartorius is the longest muscle in the body. The sartorius is attached to the front of the ilium, crosses over the medial side of the thigh and from the knee to the front of the tibia. Although it is an anterior muscle, it inserts into the tibia from behind the knee and flexes the foreleg. It also flexes, abducts, and laterally rotates the thigh at the hip. The more survivors, caregivers, and professionals know about the muscles of the body and the movements they perform, the better chance they have of strengthening the body appropriately to help in further and stronger recovery.

Did you know that having any or all of these muscles tight or the fascia locked up around these muscles can add to shoulder, hip, knee, foot, and back pain as well as add to movement issues?

Remember the fascia? It intertwines through the whole body. Fascia anywhere in the body being tight, locked up, or stuck (many ways to describe it) can cause havoc, causing pain and/or limiting movement somewhere else in the body.

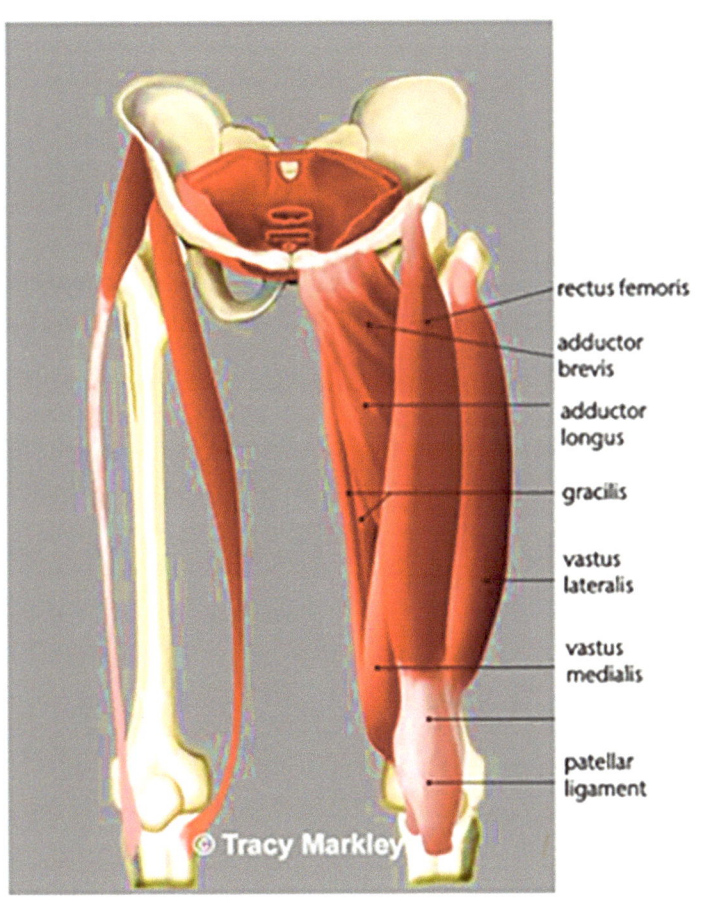

rectus femoris

adductor brevis

adductor longus

gracilis

vastus lateralis

vastus medialis

patellar ligament

© Tracy Markley

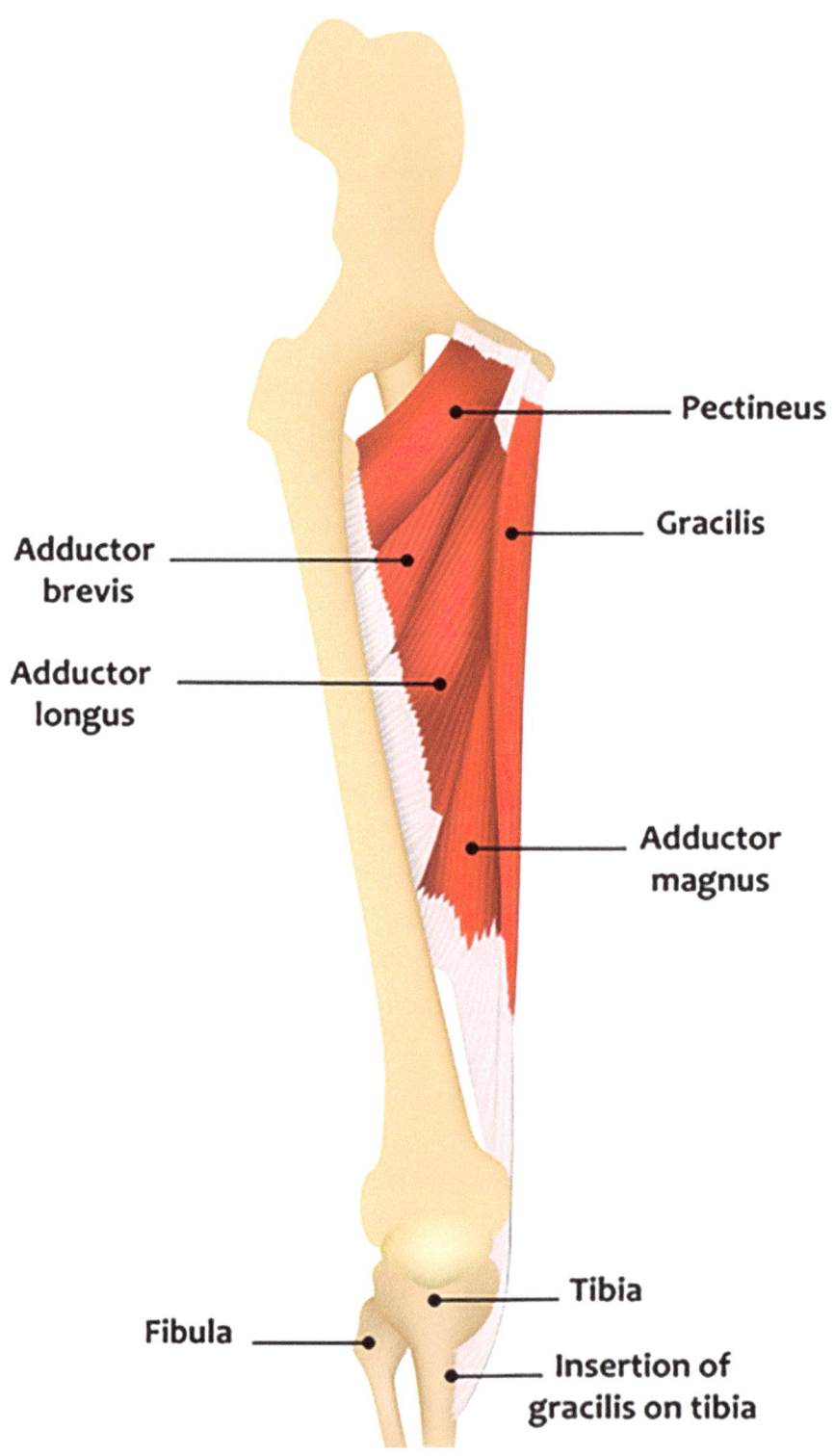

Pectineus

Gracilis

Adductor
brevis

Adductor
longus

Adductor
magnus

Tibia

Fibula

Insertion of
gracilis on tibia

Pectineus attaches to the pubis and to the femur.

It flexes the femur.

Gracilis attaches to the pubis, behind the knee and the front of the tibia. It adducts the femur.

Adductor Magnus attaches to the pubis, ischium, and the back of the femur.

Adductor Brevis attaches to the pubis and femur. It adducts the femur.

Adductor Longus attaches to the pubis and the femur. It adducts the femur.

Adductor Minimus (NOT shown in illustration) It attaches to the pubis and the femur. It adducts the femur.

All adductor muscles in the thighs pull the legs toward the middle of the body when walking. This helps maintain balance.

See my books:

Tipping Toward Balance, A Fitness Trainer's Guide to Walking, by Tracy L. Markley This book includes eight exercises that help with balance and walking.

Stroke Recovery, What Now, When Physical Therapy Ends, But Your Recovery Continues, by Tracy L. Markley. This book includes several exercises for walking, balance, back strength, posture, and stroke recovery.

Hamstrings

The back of the leg muscles

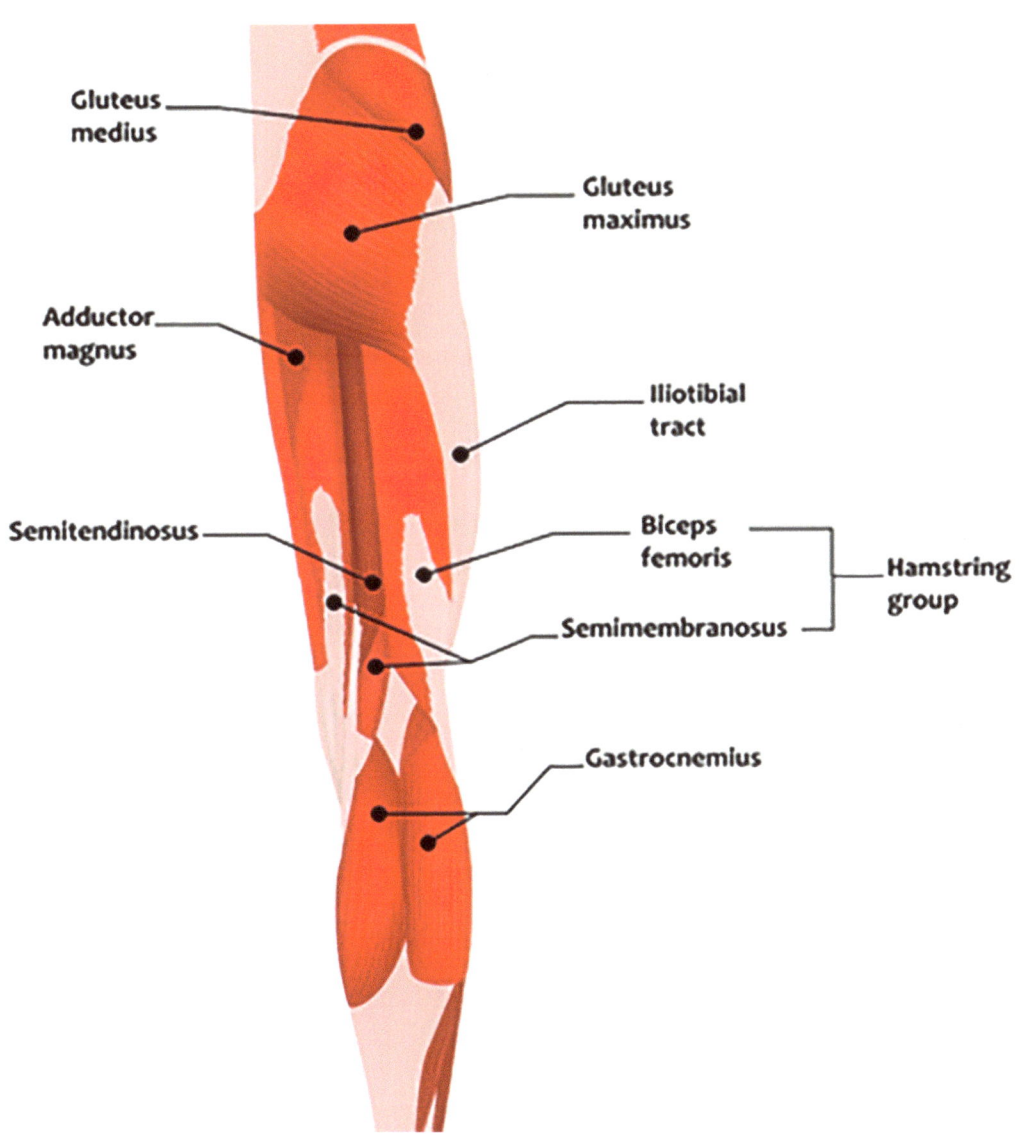

Hamstrings

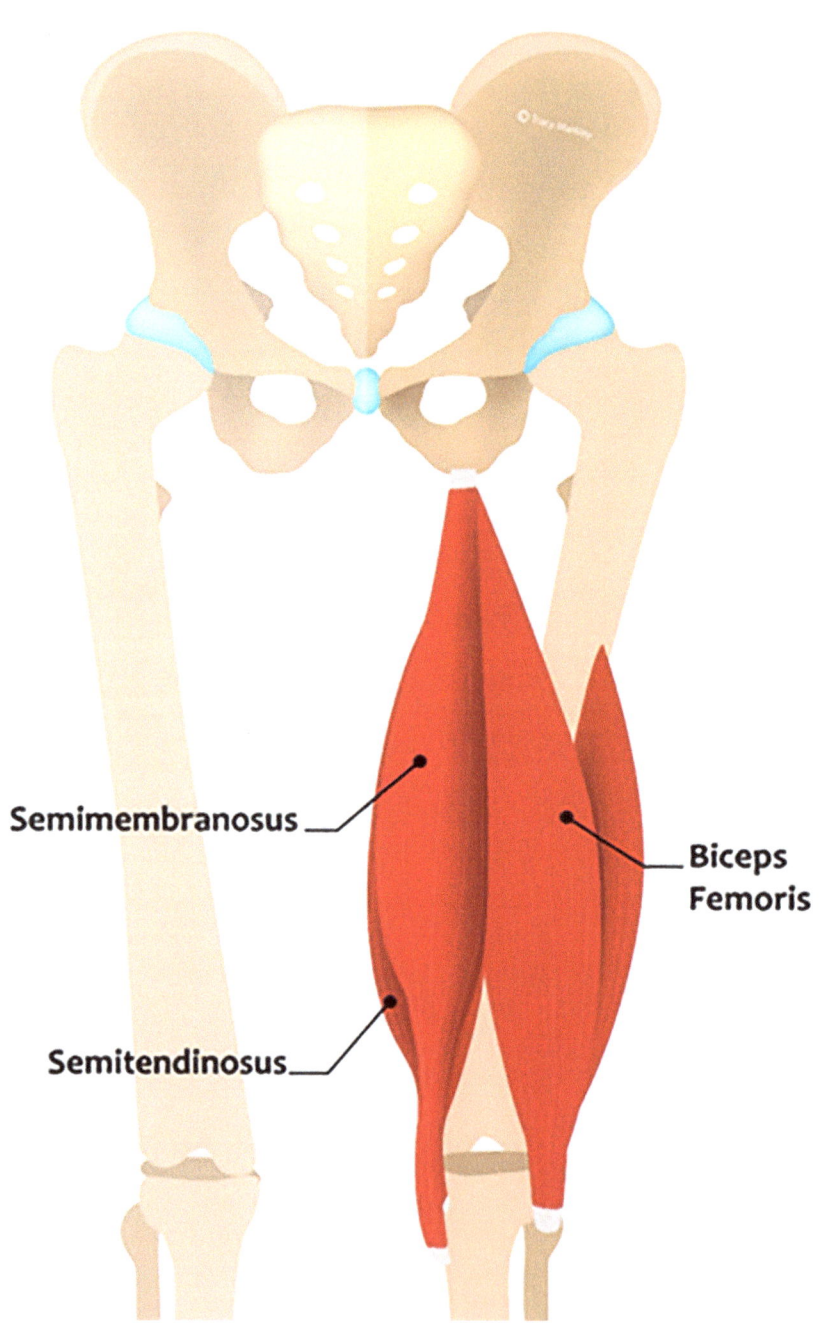

Semimembranosus

Biceps Femoris

Semitendinosus

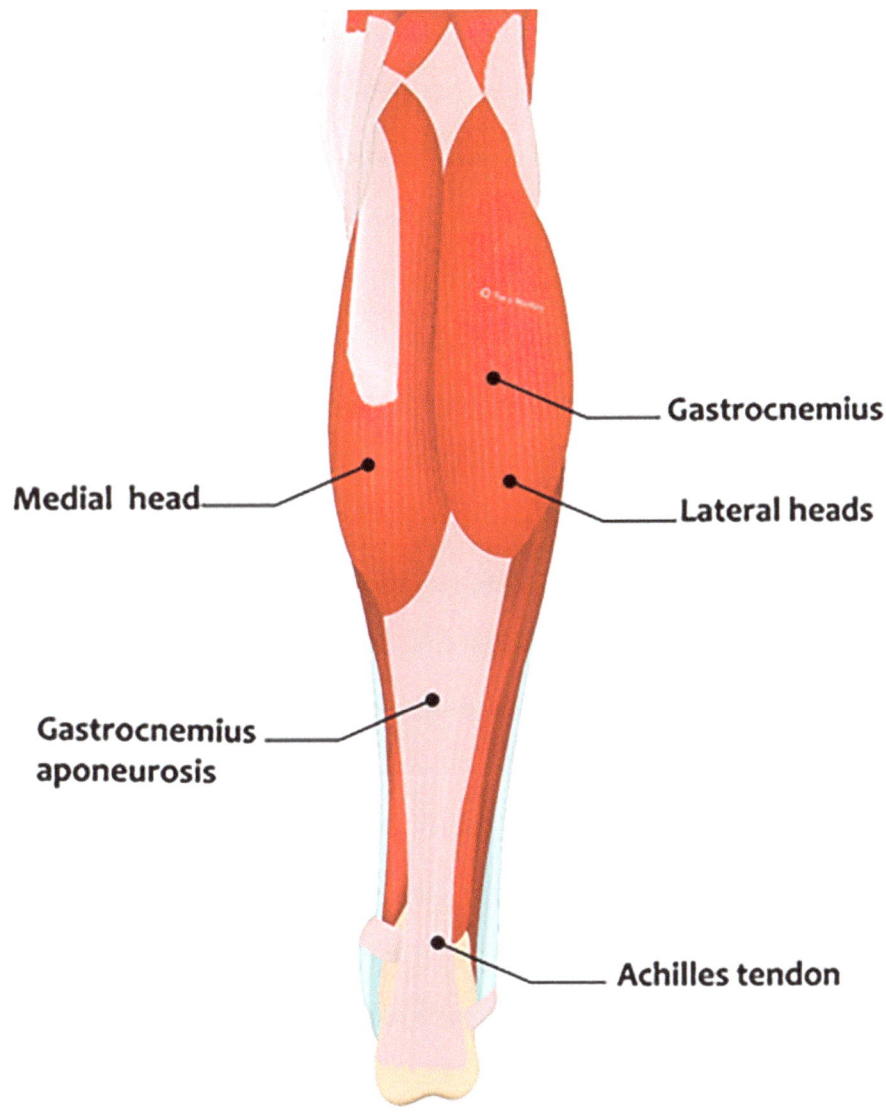

Did you know that having tight calves can add to shoulder, hip, and back pain as well as add to movement issues? Remember the fascia? It intertwines through the whole body.

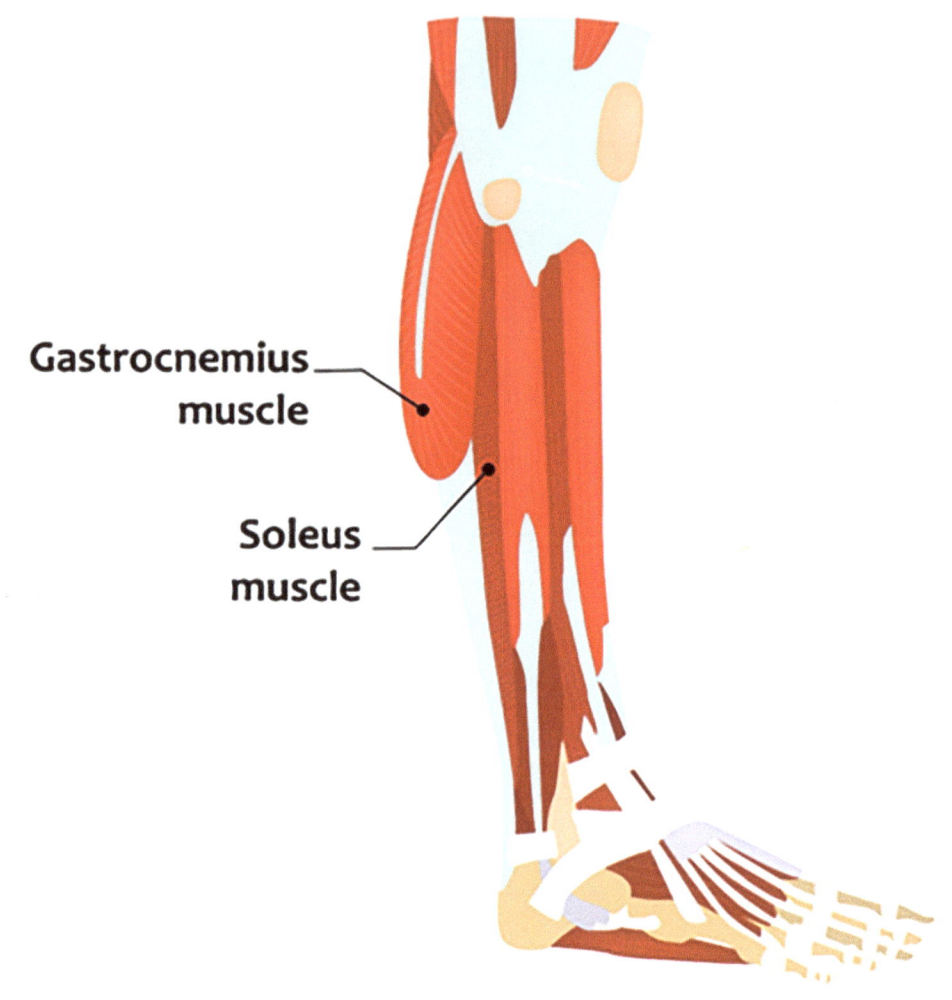

Gastrocnemius muscle

Soleus muscle

The muscles in the front of the lower leg can also add to shoulder, hip, and back pain as well as add to movement issues, if they are tight.

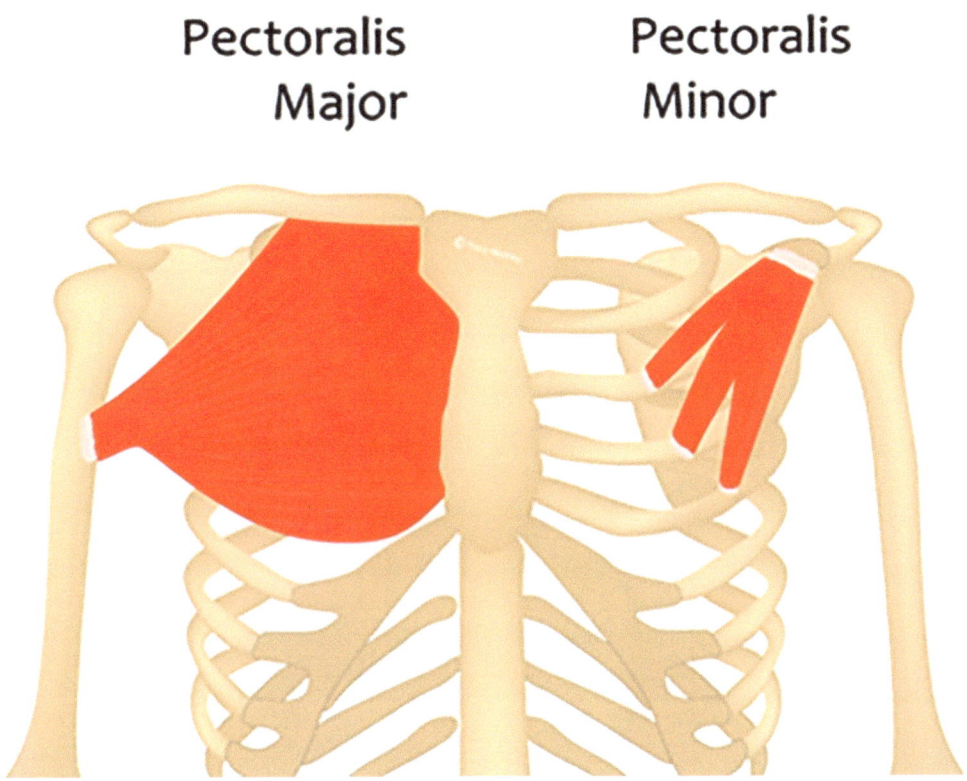

Tight chest muscles can round the shoulders forward, affecting posture, spine fascia and muscles all the way down the spine. Holding the shoulder girdle in a poor position, a malfunctioning position, can lead to bone spurs, and injuries in shoulders back and neck. Poor posture will affect many things throughout the body.

Biceps and Triceps

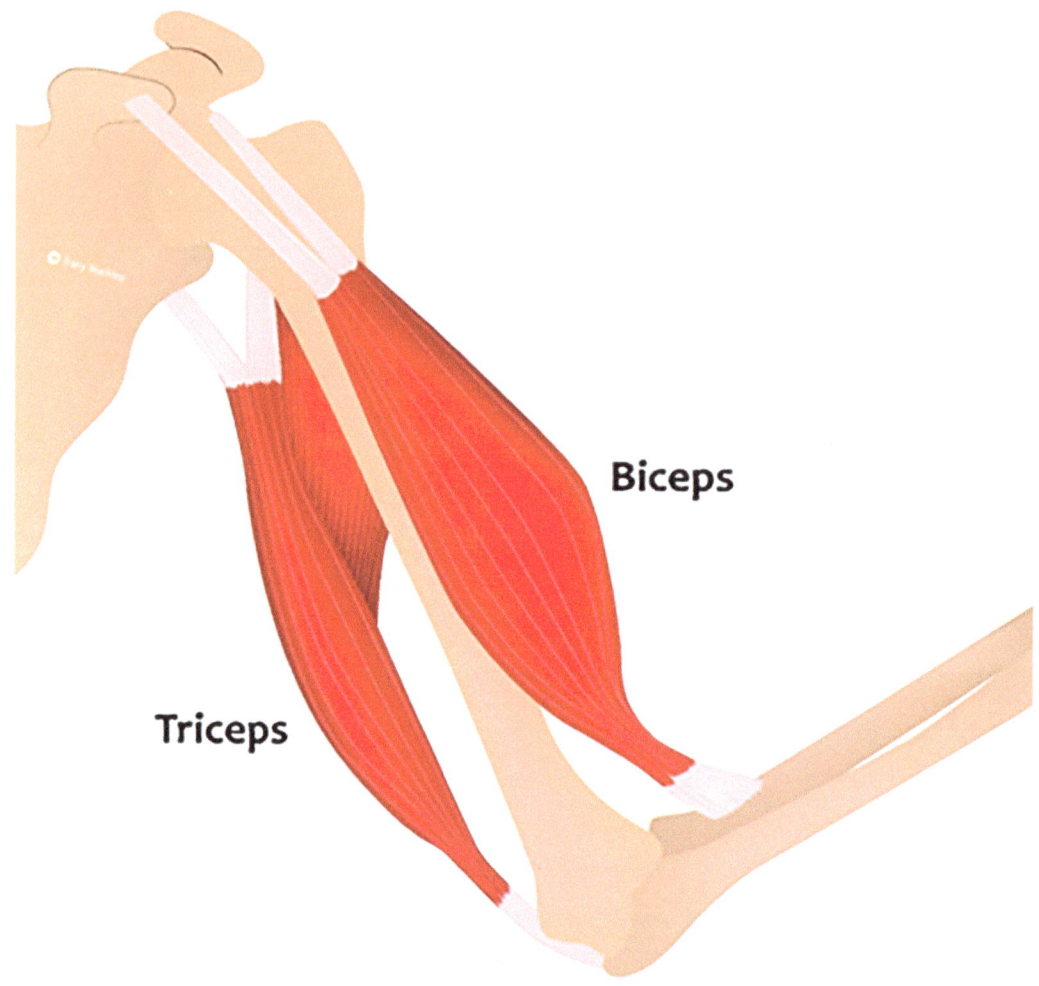

Biceps attaches at the scapula, humerus, and radius. It flexes the forearm and bends the elbow.

Triceps attaches at the scapula, humerus, and ulna. It extends the forearm and straightens the elbow.

Extra note:

Notice both the biceps and triceps attach at the scapula (shoulder blade). Biceps means two heads and Triceps means three heads.

I am also a certified yoga instructor and have taught it for years. I often have had clients come to me wanting to begin yoga because a doctor told them to try it. When this happens, I always ask the client what the doctor wants him/her to gain from taking yoga. Sometimes the answer is to gain flexibility, and sometimes, they say for their back care. We then discuss more in detail as to what is happening with each client's body/back.

In many cases, I will tell them that yoga is not the best way to heal their specific back injuries. I shared many small deep spine muscles in this book and these muscles often need to be strengthened before clients attempt to hold themselves in poses with their spine bent, flexed, twisted, and or extended. Although yoga can be great for many, it is not the fix-all to back and core muscle repair and strengthening.

Also, keep in mind there are many forms of yoga and each instructor teaches their yoga a bit differently. A qualified yoga instructor usually holds a certification that required hundreds of hours to obtain.

Pilates can be a very good modality to help heal and strengthen the spine and core, but not all Pilates is the same. Originally, "Pilates" was patented by Joseph Pilates. Several years after Joseph Pilates passed away, a group of fitness individuals took the name to court to get the patent released, so the name became generic like yoga. Not all Pilates classes and instructors teach from the Joseph Pilates method. Like yoga, a qualified Pilates instructor usually holds a certification that required hundreds of hours to obtain.

If you are looking for a fitness professional to help you gain a strong spine, back, and core to help your whole body gain functional health and rehabilitation, be sure they have some knowledge of what you have learned in this book.

Each client I work with is different, but I often use Bosu® balls, balance discs, and balance pads as well as other exercise tools. I use these when training and in rehab to gently build from the spine out and help create a healthy functioning, balanced body with good posture.

Refer to my books *Tipping Toward Balance, A Fitness Trainer's Guide to Stability and Walking* and *Stroke Recovery What Now? When Physical Therapy Ends, But Your Recovery Continues*, for exercises that strengthen the spine and core.

NOTES

HELPFUL DEFINITIONS

Anterior Towards the front of the body.

Posterior Towards the back of the body.

Superior Towards the Top of the body (above the other).

Inferior Towards the Bottom of the body (below the other).

Anatomy is the branch of science concerned with the bodily structure of humans, animals, and other living organisms, especially as revealed by dissection and the separation of parts.

Abduct When the movement is moving away from the midline of the body.

Adduct When the movement is moving toward the midline of the body.

Medial Middle

Lateral Side

Flexion A movement where two joints come together. Example: When lifting weight in a bicep curl and the elbow bends. Flexing the arm.

Extension A movement where two joints move farther apart. Example: You're in the bicep curl position with the elbow bent and you are now straightening the arm.

Knowledge Information, facts and skills acquired by a person through experience or education; the theoretical or practical understanding of a subject. Having awareness.

Awareness Knowledge or perception of a situation or fact.

Theory A supposition or a system of ideas intended to explain something.

Physiological A branch of biology that deals with the normal functions of living organisms and their parts and how they function.

Bones Hard whitish tissue making up the skeleton in humans and other vertebrates.

Joints A structure in the human or animal body at which two parts of the skeleton are joined.

NOTES

ABOUT THE AUTHOR

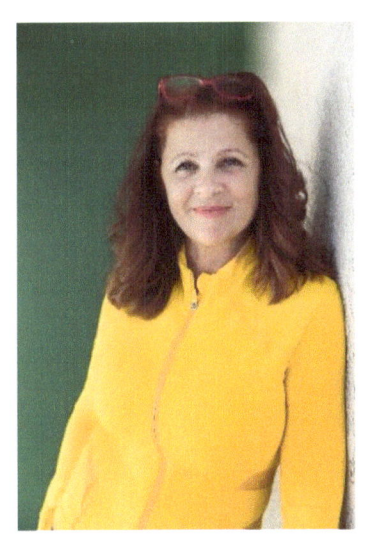

Tracy L. Markley is an award-winning author of fourteen books. She is the author and teacher of fitness education CEC courses. She was recognized by the National Fitness Hall of Fame as one of the 2024 Americas Top Fitness Educators. Her books and videos have helped stroke survivors and caregivers worldwide.

Tracy has been working and studying in the fitness industry for over 20 years. She has owned fitness studios in Oregon and California. She was the recipient of the 2021 IDEA Personal Trainer of the Year award and was one of the three finalists for the 2020 IDEA Personal Trainer of the Year award. She is a Certified Health & Fitness Specialist, Personal Trainer, Dance & Group Exercise Leader, Fitness & Nutrition, Biomechanics Specialist, BOSU® Master Trainer, AFAA Group Fitness, FiTOUR Pro- Trainer, Reiki Master-Teacher, as well as a Pilates and 200 RYT Yoga Instructor.

In 2020 Tracy was awarded the second place Medical Fitness Professional of the Year Award with the Medift Foundation. She received over twenty book awards for her books.

She has been in several magazine articles and has written fitness articles for the different newspapers. She was the host of the radio show, *The Health, and Fitness Show with Tracy* on KXCR FM radio on the Oregon Coast and she has continued the show on a podcast. She also writes a monthly article for the Live, Love, and Eat Magazine.

Tracy is available for speaking events, book signings and training. She can be contacted at her websites
www.tracymarkley.com
www.instagram.com/motivate_healthyfit
YouTube Channel: Tracy L. Markley Fitness

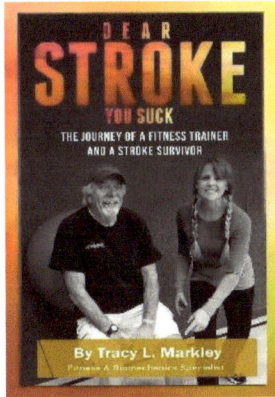
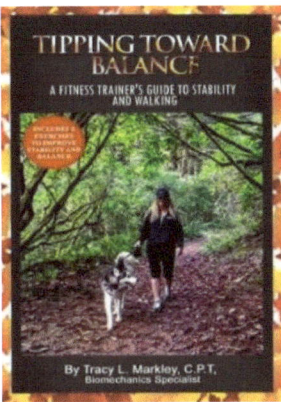
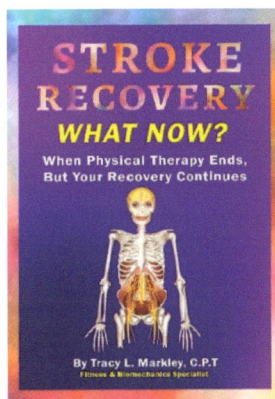
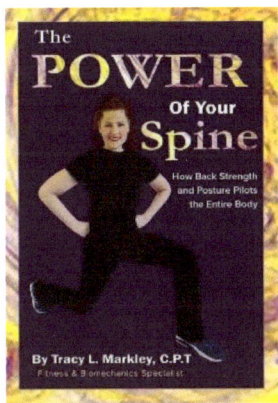
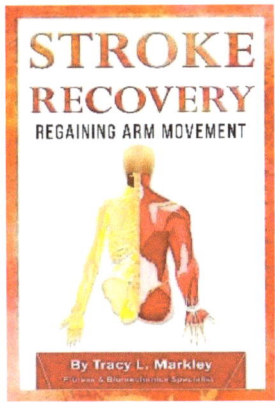
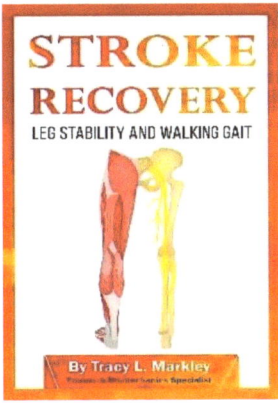
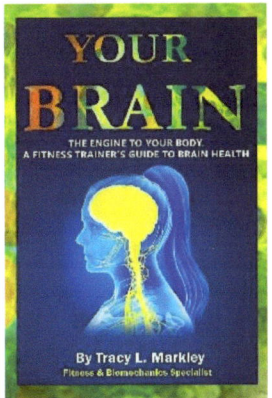
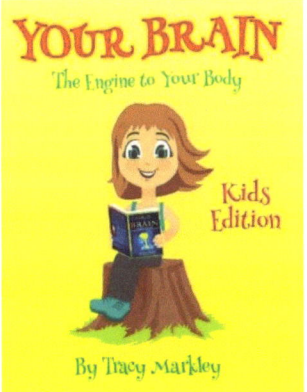
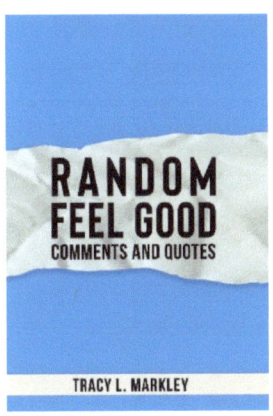
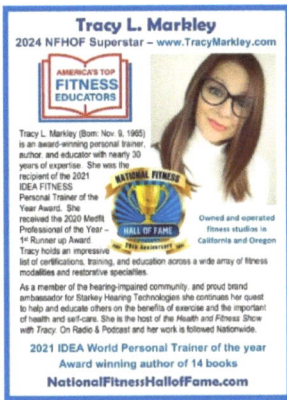
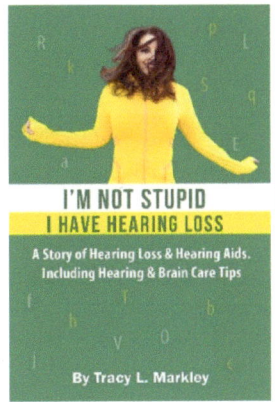
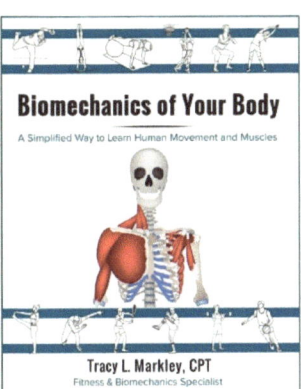

Books can be purchased at her websites or at Amazon at

www.amazon.com/author/tracymarkley

**Be kind to yourself and
never give up.
Remember the body was
made to move,
so move and exercise
it every day!**

REFERENCES

Kinesiology for the Public Schools; by J.A. Mastropaolo, 4th Edition.

Stroke Recovery, What Now, When Physical Therapy Ends, But Your Recovery Continues; by Tracy L. Markley.

Tipping Toward Balance, A Fitness Trainer's Guide to Stability and Walking; by Tracy L. Markley.

Cover Design by:
Tracy L. Markey & Oyekola Sodiq Ajibola.

Anatomy Illustrations by:
Mileidy Fernandez & Susan Lyons.

NOTES

NOTES

NOTES

www.ingramcontent.com/pod-product-compliance
Lightning Source LLC
Chambersburg PA
CBHW042027230526
45474CB00006B/30